Nicolas Goossens, Sophie Clément,
Francesco Negro

Handbook of Hepatitis C

Nicolas Goossens, Sophie Clément,
Francesco Negro

Handbook of Hepatitis C

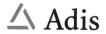 Adis

Nicolas Goossens
Division of Liver Diseases
Department of Medicine
Liver Cancer Program
Tisch Cancer Institute
Icahn School of Medicine at Mount Sinai
New York, USA
Division of Gastroenterology and Hepatology
Geneva University Hospital
Geneva, Switzerland

Sophie Clément
Clinical Pathology
University Hospitals and Faculty of Medicine
Geneva, Switzerland

Francesco Negro
Division of Gastroenterology and Hepatology
and Clinical Pathology
Geneva University Hospital
Geneva, Switzerland

ISBN 978-3-319-28051-6   ISBN (eBook) 978-3-319-28053-0
DOI 10.1007/978-3-319-28053-0
© Springer International Publishing Switzerland 2016

Printed on acid-free paper

This Adis imprint is published by Springer Nature
The registered company is AG Switzerland

Project editor: Mia Cahill

Contents

Author biographies

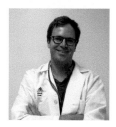

Nicolas Goossens, MD, MSc, is resident in Gastroenterology and Hepatology at the Division of Gastroenterology and Hepatology at the Geneva University Hospitals, Switzerland. He is currently research fellow at the Division of Liver Diseases under the guidance of Professor Scott Friedman and Professor Yujin Hoshida at the Mount Sinai Hospital in New York, US.

Dr Goossens earned his medical degree in 2005 from Geneva University. After training in Geneva and at the Liver Unit at the King's College Hospital in London, UK, he was board certified by the Swiss Medical Federation in Gastroenterology and then Hepatology in 2013 and 2014, respectively. Dr Goossens earned his MSc in Clinical Evidence Based Health Care from Oxford University, UK.

During his current research fellowship in New York, Dr Goossens has focused on the genomic aspects of liver diseases, in particular metabolic liver disease, hepatocellular carcinoma, and chronic hepatitis C. Dr Goossens has authored and co-authored more than 20 peer-reviewed manuscripts and reviews in the field of hepatology and gastrointestinal disease.

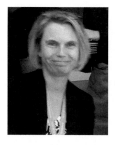

Sophie Clément, MD, PhD, currently works at the Division of Clinical Pathology of the Geneva University Hospitals, Switzerland. In 2005, she joined the Viropathology Unit, headed by Professor Francesco Negro, in the capacity of senior scientist in charge of supervising the different research projects of the laboratory.

Dr Clément obtained her PhD degree in Human Sciences from the University Claude Bernard in Lyon, France in 1995. After 2 years of post-doctoral training at Northwestern University of Chicago, US, she joined the laboratory directed by Professor Giulio Gabbiani at the Faculty of

Medicine, University of Geneva, mainly focusing her interest on myofibroblast differentiation and fibrosis.

Since she joined the laboratory of Professor Negro, she has mainly been involved in projects focusing on the metabolic disorders associated with hepatitis C virus infection, and more specifically on the mechanisms leading to insulin resistance and steatosis. She has published 25 peer-reviewed journal articles in the hepatology and hepatitis field as either first author or co-author.

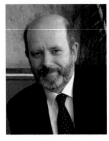 **Francesco Negro, MD,** is Professor at the Departments of Specialty Medicine and of Pathology and Immunology of the University of Geneva, Switzerland. He is also Founder and Chairman of the Swiss Hepatitis C Cohort Study, and Educational Councillor of the European Association for the Study of the Liver.

Professor Negro earned his medical degree in 1982 and was board-certified in Gastroenterology in 1986 at the University of Torino, Italy. He undertook post-doctoral training at the Division of Molecular Virology and Immunology, Georgetown University, US, and at the Hepatitis Section, National Institute of Allergy and Infectious Diseases, National Institutes of Health, US, between 1986 and 1989. Professor Negro analyzed hepatitis C virus (HCV) replication at the tissue level using several distinct approaches, establishing anatomo-clinical correlations. His studies led him to associate HCV genotype 3a with a particular form of severe liver steatosis, and to analyse the mechanisms thereof.

More recently, Professor Negro's work has focused on the pathogenesis of extrahepatic manifestations associated with HCV, and, particularly, on the mechanisms leading to glucose metabolism alterations, such as insulin resistance and diabetes, and on the epidemiology of HCV. He has participated in several clinical trials in acute and chronic HCV and has authored or co-authored more than 250 peer-reviewed manuscripts in the field of hepatology.

Abbreviations

AASLD	American Association for the Study of Liver Diseases
ALT	Alanine aminotransferase
ApoB	Apolipoprotein B
APRI	AST to platelet ratio index
ARFI	Acoustic Radiation Force Impulse Imaging
AST	Aspartate aminotransferase
CDC	Centers for Disease Control and Prevention
cDC	Conventional dendritic cell
CI	Confidence interval
DAA	Direct acting antiviral
DCs	Dendritic cells
DGAT1	Diacylglycerol O-acyltransferase 1
dsRNA	Double stranded ribonucleic acid
E	Envelope protein
EASL	European Association for the Study of the Liver
ECM	Extracellular matrix
EIA	Enzyme immunoassay
EMT	Epithelial to mesenchymal transition
ER	Endoplasmic reticulum
FDA	Food and Drug Administration
FIB-4	Fibrosis-4
HALT-C	Hepatitis C Antiviral Long-term Treatment against Cirrhosis Trial
HCC	Hepatocellular carcinoma
HCV	Hepatitis C virus
HIV	Human immunodeficiency virus
HSC	Hepatic stellate cells
IDSA	Infectious Disease Society of America
IFN	Interferon
IFN-α	Interferon-alpha
IFNL3	*Interferon-lambda3*

IL	Interleukin
IPS-1	Interferon-β promoter stimulator 1
IRES	Internal ribosome entry sites
IRS-1	Insulin receptor substrate 1
ISGs	Insulin stimulated genes
KLRG1	Killer cell lectin-like receptor G1
LDL	Low-density lipoprotein
LDLR	Low-density lipoprotein receptor
LVP	Lipo-viro-particle
MAPK	Mitogen-activated protein kinase
MHC	Major histocompatibility complex
MMPs	Matrix metalloproteinases
MTTP	Microsomal triglyceride transfer protein
NANBH	Non-A, non-B hepatitis
NK	Natural killer
NS	Non-structural
OR	Odds ratio
ORF	Open reading frame
PAMPs	Pathogen-associated molecular patterns
PCT	Porphyria cutanea tarda
PD-1	Programmed death-1
pDC	Plasmacytoid dendritic cell
P-gp	Permeability glycoprotein
PI	Protease inhibitor
PPAR-α	Peroxisome proliferator-activated receptor alpha
PRR	Pattern recognition receptors
PTEN	Phosphatase and tensin homolog deleted on chromosome 10
RAV	Resistance-associated variants
Rb	Retinoblastoma
RIG-I	Retinoic acid-inducible gene-I
SNP	Single nucleotide polymorphism
SR-B1	Scavenger receptor class B type 1

SREBP-1c	Sterol regulatory element binding protein-1c
ssRNA	Single stranded ribonucleic acid
SVR	Sustained virological response
T2DM	Type 2 diabetes mellitus
TE	Transient elastography
TGF	Transforming growth factor
TIP47	Tail-interacting protein of 47 kDa
TLR-3	Toll-like receptor 3
TRIF	Toll/interleukin-1 receptor-domain-containing adapter-inducing interferon-β
UTR	Untranslated region
VLDL	Very-low-density lipoprotein

Chapter 1

Introduction

In 2014, the scientific community celebrated the 25th anniversary of the discovery of the hepatitis C virus (HCV). Since the isolation of HCV, extensive progress has been made in the field, and a growing knowledge of the virus life cycle has led to the development of potent drugs.

This handbook will focus on the HCV particle, its life cycle, clinical features of HCV disease, pathophysiology, diagnosis, management and treatment of disease, and future challenges. An overview of current knowledge on hepatitis C and up-to-date advances are covered, with the goal to assist the medical community in the management of this disease.

Historical perspective
Discovery of HCV

In the 1970s, Harvey J Alter and his collaborators described a large number of hepatitis cases that occurred after blood transfusion and proved they were due to neither hepatitis A nor hepatitis B viruses [1]. These cases of hepatitis were thus called non-A, non-B hepatitis (NANBH) for more than 10 years. The agent responsible for hepatitis C, HCV, was first isolated and described in 1989 after the extensive screening of bacterial clones derived from experimentally infected chimpanzee samples by researchers from the Chiron Corporation in California [2–4]. Since the isolation of HCV the interest in this field has expanded remarkably, as reflected by the number of publications found in PubMed using 'hepatitis C virus' as a query (Figure 1.1).

© Springer International Publishing Switzerland 2016
N. Goossens et al. (eds.), *Handbook of Hepatitis C*,
DOI 10.1007/978-3-319-28053-0_1

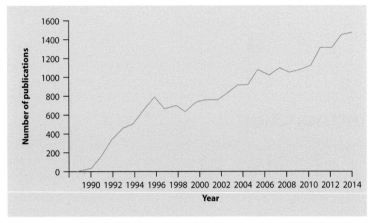

Figure 1.1 The number of publications obtained in PubMed from 1990 to 2014 when using 'hepatitis C virus' as query in the publication title.

Main scientific and medical advances in HCV research

The discovery of HCV led to the development of diagnostic tools and, in the early 1990s, the implementation of systematic screening of blood supplies; in the US this contributed to the reduction of infection via blood transfusion by almost 100% [5]. In 1991, the use of interferon-alpha (IFN-α) as a treatment for hepatitis C disease was approved and in 1998 the combination of IFN-α and ribavirin was approved. In 2001, pegylated IFN-α (peg-IFN-α) (which has improved pharmacokinetics and efficacy compared to IFN-α) was introduced. Despite the potentially severe side effects of this regimen it remained the gold standard for over 10 years; the sustained virological response (SVR) could reach up to 50% [6] in certain subgroups. During this time extensive efforts have been undertaken to develop cell culture systems, which have helped the development of direct acting antiviral (DAA) drugs (Chapter 6). The replicon system, developed in 1999, allowed a better understanding of HCV replication in the human hepatoma cell line Huh-7 [7]. Major advances in the study of HCV entry and neutralizing antibodies were achieved thanks to the establishment of the HCV pseudoparticle system in 2003, which consists of lentiviral particles harboring HCV envelope protein (E)1 and E2 [8]. The major breakthrough in HCV research has undeniably been the development of the JFH1-based cell culture system, which recapitulated the complete HCV life cycle in vitro [9] (Figure 1.2).

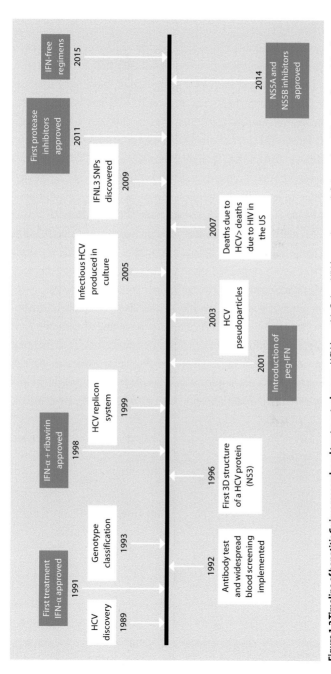

Figure 1.2 Timeline of hepatitis C virus research and treatment advances. HCV, hepatitis C virus; HIV, human immunodeficiency virus; IFN-α, interferon-alpha; IL, interleukin; NS, non-structural; peg-IFN, pegylated interferon; SNPs, single nucleotide polymorphisms.

Epidemiology

HCV infection is a major health problem worldwide. A recent study based on anti-HCV seroprevalence data estimated that 185 million people, corresponding to 2.8% of the world's population, have been infected with HCV [10]. Among those infected with HCV, the World Health Organization estimates that 130–150 million individuals worldwide are chronically infected [11]. The Centers for Disease Control and Prevention (CDC) estimates that in the US alone approximately 29,700 new cases are diagnosed per year, a number that is steadily increasing [12]. Global mortality due to hepatitis C infection is approximately 700,000 individuals per year [13]. In the US, the number of deaths from HCV was 19,368 in 2013 [12] and a large study reviewing the death certificates of 22 million deceased people demonstrated that the number of deaths due to HCV (15,106) surpassed those due to human immunodeficiency virus (HIV) infection (12,734) in 2007 [14].

HCV infection is prevalent worldwide and its geographical distribution varies (Figure 1.3). North Africa, East Asia, and the Middle East have the highest prevalence of HCV [15], estimated at more than 3.5%. Within North Africa prevalence is highest in Egypt (approximately 15%); this is thought to be a consequence of a prophylaxis campaign against schistosomiasis carried out between 1961 and 1986 [16]. By contrast,

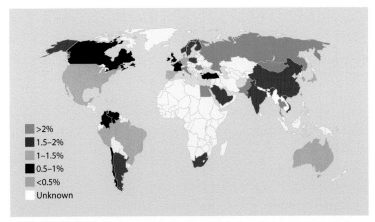

Figure 1.3 Hepatitis C virus prevalence worldwide [14]. Reproduced with permission from © John Wiley and Sons.

prevalence in industrialized countries in Europe, America, and Australia has been reported to be significantly lower, with the exception of Spain and Russia, where prevalence is 1.5 [17] and 2.9% [18], respectively, and central and south Italy and Romania where it is higher than 3% [19]. However, it should be noted that most of the prevalence data are based on specific person subgroups that are not necessarily representative of the overall population of one country. Additionally, epidemiologic data are not available in all countries. For example, in Africa robust data are only available for Egypt and South Africa.

HCV genotypes

HCV has a high capability to generate mutations and exists as seven different genotypes, subdivided into more than 60 subtypes [20]. HCV circulates within a single patient as closely related variants named 'quasispecies'. This constant variation of the HCV genome is the major reason for the difficulties encountered in the development of a vaccine against HCV. Based on nucleotide homology analysis of the non-structural (NS)5 region of the HCV genome, it has been estimated that strains from different genotypes share a similarity of between 67 and 69%. Within subtypes of HCV only 20–25% of nucleotides are different [21]. In 2015 Messina et al [22] carried out a large retrospective literature analysis combining epidemiologic data from 1217 studies published between 1989 and 2013, representing 117 countries. The study demonstrated that genotype 1 is the most predominant (42%), followed by genotype 3 (30%). The sum of genotype 2, 4, and 6 corresponds to approximately 23%, while genotype 5 represents less than 1% of the total number of HCV cases. HCV genotype 7 was first described in 2014 [20] and has been reported so far in only a few patients [23,24].

Genotype 1 is widely spread throughout the world; however, the other genotypes have more restricted geographical distributions. Genotype 2 predominates in West Africa, genotype 4 in the Middle East, genotype 5 in South Africa, and genotype 6 in East and South East Asia, and is the main genotype in Vietnam [15,22]. Although genotype 3 is widely distributed, its prevalence is particularly high in South Asia (Figure 1.4). The prevalence of genotypes and subtypes is different depending on the transmission route. For example, genotypes 1a and 3a are more frequent among intravenous drug users (63% and 33%, respectively) while genotype 1b has a high prevalence among patients who were infected through blood transfusions [25]. Although all genotypes can establish chronic infection, there are specific clinical disease features associated with genotypes; steatosis, for example, is more prevalent in genotype 3 infections [26] (see Chapter 4). The response to therapy is also dependent on HCV genotype; genotype 1 and 4 infections are the most difficult to cure with peg-IFN-α and ribavirin combination therapy as compared to genotypes 2 and 3 [27], whereas chances of SVR to IFN-free regimens appear to be lower in genotype 3-infected patients (see Chapter 6).

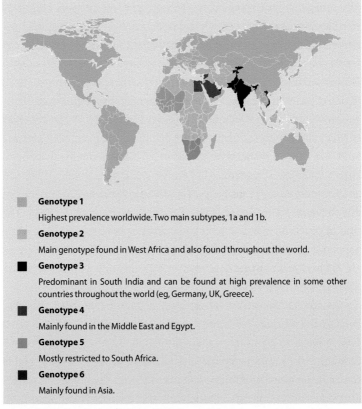

Genotype 1
Highest prevalence worldwide. Two main subtypes, 1a and 1b.

Genotype 2
Main genotype found in West Africa and also found throughout the world.

Genotype 3
Predominant in South India and can be found at high prevalence in some other countries throughout the world (eg, Germany, UK, Greece).

Genotype 4
Mainly found in the Middle East and Egypt.

Genotype 5
Mostly restricted to South Africa.

Genotype 6
Mainly found in Asia.

Figure 1.4 Hepatitis C virus genotype distribution and prevalence around the world.
Adapted from Negro and Alberti [15] and Messina et al [22].

Modes of disease transmission and risk factors

The principal route of transmission of HCV is via the blood. In developed countries, since the systematic screening of blood donors, the risk of HCV infection consecutive to transfusion or organ transplant has dramatically decreased to less than 1 per 100,000 [28]. In some countries, however, HCV can still be transmitted via the transfusion of unscreened blood. HCV was also identified to be highly present among patients receiving long-term dialysis, with a prevalence of anti-HCV positive patients in this population ranging from 1 to 70% (depending on the country) [29]. Of course, the risk of HCV transmission in patients on dialysis is largely increased by the number of transfusions and the time spent on dialysis, but once again, transmission of HCV by blood transfusions is now very rare in dialysis units of developed countries thanks to the introduction of systematic screening of blood donors and the extensive implementation of safety procedures [29]. Organ transplantation is another route of HCV transmission [30]; even though the screening of donors has been implemented in developed countries, some cases of HCV transmission due to organ transplantation are still reported [31].

Any source of blood is able to transmit the virus, even if it is indirect (such as soiled material). Tattooing, body piercing, or even acupuncture have also probably contributed to the spread of HCV, even in developed countries. In health care settings, needle-stick injuries, unsafe injections, and reuse or improper sterilization of contaminated medical equipment are also responsible for some cases of HCV infection in developed countries and still represent a major route of transmission in resource-poor areas of the world. During the year 2000, it has been estimated that 16,000 health care workers worldwide were infected by HCV following percutaneous injuries [32]. In developed countries, however, the most significant risk for HCV infection is related to intravenous drug use through the sharing of contaminated needles and other paraphernalia. This mode of transmission accounts for more than 60% of newly diagnosed cases of hepatitis C [33]. Cocaine users have also been shown to transmit the virus by sharing snorting straws [34]. HCV can be transmitted sexually, although this route of transmission is uncommon. In groups of people with high-risk sexual behavior, such as HIV-positive men who have sex with men, the incidence of HCV is higher than in the general population and has increased in recent years [35]. By contrast, in monogamous serodiscordant couples the risk of transmission is very low and has been estimated to be <0.25% per year [36–38]. One explanation for this low rate of transmission may be that seronegative partners somehow develop immune defenses against HCV via regular contact with small amounts of virus.

The vertical (mother-to-child) transmission rate is around 4% [39] and can occur both during pregnancy and at the time of the delivery. The type of delivery (vaginal versus cesarean) does not appear to impact on the risk of transmission [39]. Importantly, reports have shown that co-infection with HIV increases the risk of maternal-fetal transmission of HCV [35].

Economic and social burden

HCV infection is a major health concern worldwide due to its high prevalence and the fact that HCV-associated disease has long-term consequences. The latter is of great importance considering that over 75% of infected adults are 'baby-boomers' (a term that refers to those born between 1945 and 1965) [40] and that the burden of HCV will significantly increase over the next decade with increased projected cases of cirrhosis and hepatocellular carcinoma (HCC), despite improved cure rates for HCV. Another important issue is the low diagnosis rate, which potentially leads to an underestimation of the overall number of patients. The US CDC run a national campaign, Know More Hepatitis™, which provides information about hepatitis C and encourages people born between 1945 and 1965 to get tested [40]. With the arrival of IFN-free regimens expected SVR rates are greater than 90% but barriers to treatment access remain significant (eg, inadequate screening, poor linkage to care, and high cost of treatment) and many people remain untreated [41]. If we take into account the indirect costs of untreated chronic HCV (absenteeism and lower work productivity of HCV-infected individuals [42]), treating HCV with efficacious drugs is certainly cost-effective in most subgroups of patients [43].

Key points

- Between 130 and 180 million people are infected with HCV worldwide and there are around 700,000 deaths related to HCV per year.
- Prevalence is highest in Africa and Asia and lowest in North America, Europe, and Australia.
- Risk factors include intravenous drug use, co-infection with HIV, history of blood transfusion or organ transplant before 1992, history of long-term hemodialysis, history of detention, and tattoos or body piercings.
- Route of transmission is mainly via blood (syringe exchange between drug users, transfusion of unscreened blood, tattoos, piercing, reuse or improper sterilization of contaminated medical equipment, and needle-stick injuries).
- Mother-to-baby transmission can occur (especially if the mother is co-infected with HIV).
- Sexual transmission is rare.

References

1   Feinstone SM, Kapikian AZ, Purcell RH, Alter HJ, Holland PV. Transfusion-associated hepatitis not due to viral hepatitis type A or B. *N Engl J Med.* 1975;292:767–770.

2   Alter HJ, Purcell RH, Shih JW, et al. Detection of antibody to hepatitis C virus in prospectively followed transfusion recipients with acute and chronic non-A, non-B hepatitis. *N Engl J Med.* 1989; 321:1494–500.

3   Choo QL, Kuo G, Weiner AJ, Overby LR, Bradley DW, Houghton M. Isolation of a cDNA clone derived from a blood-borne non-A, non-B viral hepatitis genome. Science. 1989;244:359–362.

4   Houghton M. Discovery of the hepatitis C virus. *Liver Int.* 2009;29 (Suppl 1) :82–88.

5   Selvarajah S, Busch MP. Transfusion transmission of HCV, a long but successful road map to safety. *Antivir Ther.* 2012;17:1423–1429.

6   Dienstag JL, McHutchison JG. American Gastroenterological Association technical review on the management of hepatitis C. *Gastroenterology.* 2006;130:231–264.

7   Lohmann V, Körner F, Koch J, Herian U, Theilmann L, Bartenschlager R. Replication of subgenomic hepatitis C virus RNAs in a hepatoma cell line. *Science.* 1999;285:110–113.

8   Bartosch B, Dubuisson J, Cosset FL. Infectious hepatitis C virus pseudo-particles containing functional E1-E2 envelope protein complexes. *J Exp Med.* 2003;197:633–642.

9   Wakita T, Pietschmann T, Kato T, et al. Production of infectious hepatitis C virus in tissue culture from a cloned viral genome. *Nat Med.* 2005;11:791–796.

10 Mohd Hanafiah K, Groeger J, Flaxman AD, Wiersma ST, et al. Global epidemiology of hepatitis C virus infection: new estimates of age-specific antibody to HCV seroprevalence. *Hepatology.* 2013;57:1333–1342.

11   World Health Organization. Hepatitis C. Fact sheet N° 164. Available at: www.who.int/mediacentre/factsheets/fs164/en/ (2015). Accessed 27 Nov 2015.

12   Centers for Disease Control and Prevention. Viral Hepatitis - Statistics and Surveillance. Disease Burden from Viral Hepatitis A, B, and C in the United States. Available at: www.cdc.gov/hepatitis/Statistics/index.htm (2013). Accessed 27 Nov 2015.

13   GBD 2013 Mortality and Causes of Death Collaborators. Global, regional, and national age-sex specific all-cause and cause-specific mortality for 240 causes of death, 1990–2013: a systematic analysis for the Global Burden of Disease Study 2013. *Lancet*. 2015;385:117–171.

14   Ly KN, Xing J, Klevens RM, Jiles RB, Ward JW, Holmberg SD. The increasing burden of mortality from viral hepatitis in the United States between 1999 and 2007. *Ann Intern Med*. 2012;156:271–278.

15   Negro F, Alberti A. The global health burden of hepatitis C virus infection. *Liver Int*. 2011;31 (Suppl 2):1–3.

16   Frank C, Mohamed MK, Strickland GT, et al. The role of parenteral antischistosomal therapy in the spread of hepatitis C virus in Egypt. *Lancet*. 2000;355:887–891.

17   Bruggmann P, Berg T, Øvrehus AL, et al. Historical epidemiology of hepatitis C virus (HCV) in selected countries. *J Viral Hepat*. 2014;21 (Suppl 1):5–33.

18   Saraswat V, Norris S, de Knegt RJ, et al. Historical epidemiology of hepatitis C virus (HCV) in select countries - volume 2. *J Viral Hepat*. 2015;22 (Suppl 1):6–25.

19   Cornberg M, Razavi HA, Alberti A, et al. A systematic review of hepatitis C virus epidemiology in Europe, Canada and Israel. *Liver Int*. 2011l;31 (Suppl 2):30–60.

20   Smith DB, Bukh J, Kuiken C, et al. Expanded classification of hepatitis C virus into 7 genotypes and 67 subtypes: updated criteria and genotype assignment web resource. *Hepatology*. 2014;59:318–327.

21   Simmonds P, Bukh J, Combet C, et al. Consensus proposals for a unified system of nomenclature of hepatitis C virus genotypes. *Hepatology*. 2005;42:962–973.

22   Messina JP, Humphreys I, Flaxman A, et al. Global distribution and prevalence of hepatitis C virus genotypes. *Hepatology*. 2015;61:77–87.

23   Murphy DG, Sablon E, Chamberland J, Fournier E, Dandavino R, Tremblay CL, et al. Hepatitis C virus genotype 7, a new genotype originating from central Africa. *J Clin Microbiol*. 2015;53:967–972.

24   Murphy DG, Willems B, Deschênes M, Hilzenrat N, Mousseau R, Sabbah S. Use of sequence analysis of the NS5B region for routine genotyping of hepatitis C virus with reference to C/E1 and 5' untranslated region sequences. *J Clin Microbiol*. 2007;45:1102–1112.

25   Pawlotsky JM, Tsakiris L, Roudot-Thoraval F, et al. Relationship between hepatitis C virus genotypes and sources of infection in patients with chronic hepatitis C. *J Infect Dis*. 1995;171:1607–1610.

26   Rubbia-Brandt L, Fabris P, Paganin S, et al. Steatosis affects chronic hepatitis C progression in a genotype specific way. *Gut*. 2004;53:406–412.

27   Wohnsland A, Hofmann WP, Sarrazin C. Viral determinants of resistance to treatment in patients with hepatitis C. *Clin Microbiol Rev*. 2007;20:23–38.

28   Alter HJ, Houghton M. Clinical Medical Research Award. Hepatitis C virus and eliminating post-transfusion hepatitis. *Nat Med*. 2000;6:1082–1086.

29   Fabrizi F. Hepatitis C virus infection and dialysis: 2012 update. *ISRN Nephrol*. 2012;2013:159760.

30   Pereira BJ, Milford EL, Kirkman RL, Levey AS. Transmission of hepatitis C virus by organ transplantation. *N Engl J Med*. 1991;325:454–460.

31   Ellingson K, Seem D, Nowicki M, Strong DM, Kuehnert MJ; Organ Procurement Organization Nucleic Acid Testing Yield Project Team. Estimated risk of human immunodeficiency virus and hepatitis C virus infection among potential organ donors from 17 organ procurement organizations in the United States. *Am J Transplant*. 2011;11:1201–1208.

32   Prüss-Ustün A, Rapiti E, Hutin Y. Estimation of the global burden of disease attributable to contaminated sharps injuries among health-care workers. *Am J Ind Med*. 2005;48:482–490.

33 Wiessing L, Guarita B, Giraudon I, Brummer-Korvenkontio H, Salminen M, Cowan SA. European monitoring of notifications of hepatitis C virus infection in the general population among injecting drug users (IDUs) - the need to improve quality and comparability. *Euro Surveill*. 2008;13:18884.

34 Harsch HH, Pankiewicz J, Bloom AS, et al. Hepatitis C virus infection in cocaine users--a silent epidemic. *Community Ment Health J*. 2000;36:225–233.

35 Wandeler G, Gsponer T, Bregenzer A, et al. Hepatitis C virus infections in the Swiss HIV Cohort Study: a rapidly evolving epidemic. *Clin Infect Dis*. 2012;55:1408–1416.

36 Terrault NA, Dodge JL, Murphy EL, et al. Sexual transmission of hepatitis C virus among monogamous heterosexual couples: the HCV partners study. *Hepatology*. 2013;57:881–889.

37 Vandelli C, Renzo F, Romanò L, et al. Lack of evidence of sexual transmission of hepatitis C among monogamous couples: results of a 10-year prospective follow-up study. *Am J Gastroenterol*. 2004;99:855–859.

38 Kao JH, Liu CJ, Chen PJ, Chen W, Lai MY, Chen DS. Low incidence of hepatitis C virus transmission between spouses: a prospective study. *J Gastroenterol Hepatol*. 2000;15:391–395.

39 Yeung LT, King SM, Roberts EA. Mother-to-infant transmission of hepatitis C virus. *Hepatology*. 2001;34:223–229.

40 US Department of Health and Human Services. Centers for Disease Control and Prevention. Hepatitis C. Why Baby Boomers should get tested. Publication No. 220401. Avaiblable at www.cdc.gov/knowmorehepatitis/Media/PDFs/FactSheet-Boomers.pdf (2015). Accessed 28 Jan 2016.

41 Economic Intelligence Unit. The Silent Pandemic: Tackling Hepatitis C with Policy Innovation. A report from the Economist Intelligence Unit. Available at: www.janssen.ie/sites/stage-janssen-ie.emea.cl.datapipe.net/files/The%20Silent%20Pandemic%20-%20Tackling%20Hepatitis%20C%20with%20Policy%20Innovation.pdf (2012). Accessed 27 Nov 2015.

42 Su J, Brook RA, Kleinman NL, Corey-Lisle P. The impact of hepatitis C virus infection on work absence, productivity, and healthcare benefit costs. *Hepatology*. 2010;52:436–442.

43 Estes C, Abdel-Kareem M, Abdel-Razek W, et al. Economic burden of hepatitis C in Egypt: the future impact of highly effective therapies. *Aliment Pharmacol Ther*. 2015;42:696–706.

Chapter 2

The HCV particle and its life cycle

The HCV particle

The hepatitis C virus (HCV) belongs to the *Hepacivirus* genus of the *Flaviviridae* family of viruses. HCV is an enveloped, positive-strand RNA virus that is spherical and has a diameter of between 40 and 80 nm in HCV-infected patients [1] and between 60 and 75 nm in cell culture systems [2]. It is composed of an envelope (derived from host cell membranes), two viral glycoproteins, envelope proteins (E)1 and E2, and an icosahedral capsid containing a positive-sense, single-stranded RNA genome (Figure 2.1). The HCV RNA genome is 9.6 kb in length [3], flanked by 5' and 3' untranslated regions (UTR), and contains two open reading frames (ORF). The large ORF encodes the entire HCV polyprotein and the alternative ORF produces a single protein, the F protein [4]. The role of the F protein is not well understood, although it has been suggested that it could be implicated in immune evasion [5]. The 5'UTR is highly conserved among different HCV isolates and the secondary structure contains four distinct stem-loops called internal ribosome entry sites (IRES) that are essential for the cap-independent translation of the genomic RNA [6]. The 3'UTR contains a variable region, followed by a poly-U/UC and 3'X region. Mechanisms underlying the functional roles of the 3'UTR region are unclear; nevertheless, a recent study has shown that the 3'UTR may enhance translation by transferring the host translation machinery components from the 3' to the 5' end of viral RNA [7].

© Springer International Publishing Switzerland 2016
N. Goossens et al. (eds.), *Handbook of Hepatitis C*,
DOI 10.1007/978-3-319-28053-0_2

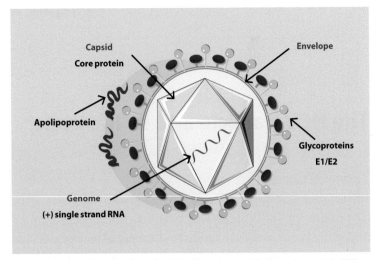

Figure 2.1 The structure of the hepatitis C virus lipo-viro-particle. E, envelope protein; RNA, ribonucleic acid. This figure was produced using Servier Medical Art, available from www.servier.com/Powerpoint-image-bank.

A unique aspect of HCV is that it is found in the blood in the form of lipo-viro-particles (LVP), which contain low-density lipoprotein (LDL) and very-low-density lipoprotein (VLDL) components (eg, apolipoproteins E and B, and triglycerides) that surround the particle [8]. Although the precise role of LVP formation remains unclear, it seems that it plays a role in HCV entry (as HCV particles use receptors implicated in lipid uptake [see below section]) and in immune escape (as lipoproteins surrounding HCV particles potentially protect them from neutralizing antibody recognition) [8].

The HCV life cycle

The elucidation of the HCV life cycle has proven to have many important implications in the development of novel anti-HCV molecules, and therefore the following section will provide the most relevant information on the different steps of the viral life cycle (Figure 2.2).

Entry into the cell

The first step in the HCV life cycle is attachment to and entry into host cells. HCV has a restricted tropism, infecting predominantly hepatocytes,

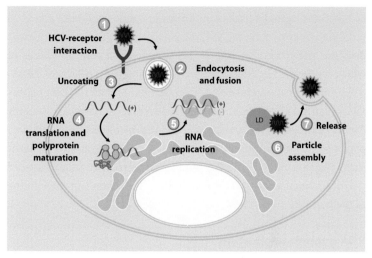

Figure 2.2 Schematic representation of the hepatitis C virus life cycle. The seven steps of the life cycle are depicted: 1, attachment; 2, entry by endocytosis and fusion; 3, uncoating; 4, RNA translation and polyprotein maturation; 5, RNA replication; 6, particle assembly on lipid droplets; and 7, release. HCV, hepatitis C virus; LD, lipid; RNA, ribonucleic acid. This figure was produced using Servier Medical Art, available from www.servier.com/Powerpoint-image-bank.

explaining the liver disorders induced by HCV infection. The process of HCV entry is meticulously orchestrated and involves many cellular receptors. First, the LVP binds to glycosaminoglycans, LDL receptor (LDLR) [9], and scavenger receptor class B type 1 (SR-B1) [10]. The interaction of HCV with SR-B1 then induces conformational changes of the viral envelope glycoprotein E2, leading to the binding of E2 to the tetraspanin CD81 [11]. CD81 and tight junction proteins (occludin and claudin-1) form a complex that triggers HCV to be internalized by clathrin-mediated endocytosis [12]. The low pH within the endosomal compartment induces major conformational changes of the E1 glycoprotein, leading to membrane fusion and capsid release into the cytoplasm.

RNA genome translation and protein maturation

Upon decapsidation the HCV genome is released into the cytoplasm of the host cell, where it is considered by the cellular machinery as mRNA, and is therefore directly translated. The cellular ribosomes recognize the IRES at the 5'UTR and produce a polyprotein, which is then cleaved by cellular host (signal peptidase and signal peptide peptidase) and viral proteases (non-structural [NS]2-NS3 and NS3-NS4) into ten distinct proteins: the structural and the NS proteins, the main functions of which are detailed in Table 2.1. Several host and viral (NS2, NS3, NS4A, NS4B) factors can modulate HCV translation. Among the host factors the human autoantigen, La, has been shown to favor ribosome assembly during initiation of translation [13] and the microRNA, miR-122, also play a major role in activating translation by targeting two adjacent sites upstream of the HCV IRES [14,15]. Translation and maturation of the viral proteins occur at the endoplasmic reticulum (ER) membrane of the host cell.

RNA genome replication

Replication occurs once the amount of viral protein is sufficient. The mechanisms implicated in the switch from translation to replication are poorly understood but it has been hypothesized that NS3 and autoantigen La are involved. One such hypothesis suggests that NS3 and autoantigen La, which have antagonist effects on translation (ie, NS3 inhibits translation while autoantigen La activates it), compete for binding to IRES and

Hepatitis C virus proteins	Main known functions
Structural proteins	
Core	Capsid protein
E1	Envelope glycoprotein — fusion of the viral with cellular membranes
E2	Envelope glycoprotein — attachment to the cell
Non-structural proteins	
p7	Formation of ion channel in endoplasmic reticulum membrane
NS2	Protease — cleavage at the NS2-3 site
NS3	Protease — cleavage at the NS3/4A, NS4A/B, NS4B/5A, and NS5A/B sites
NS4A	Helicase — role in the viral RNA replication process
NS4B	Cofactor of NS3
NS5A	Formation of membranous structures essential for viral replication
NS5B	Regulation of viral replication
	RNA-dependent-RNA polymerase — replication of the hepatitis C virus genome

Table 2.1 Hepatitis C virus proteins and their main functions. E, envelope protein; NS, non-structural; RNA, ribonucleic acid.

therefore could participate in this molecular switch from translation to replication [16].

The viral protein, NS5B, is the RNA-dependent-RNA polymerase responsible for RNA replication [17]. Replication takes place in a specific membrane structure — the membranous web — the formation of which is induced by the virus itself [18] and is considered as the HCV RNA factory. NS5B replicates the positive-sense strand into a negative-sense strand intermediate that serves as a template for the synthesis of the genomic strand. Several host and viral proteins are involved in the regulation of replication. Among these, cyclophilin A and B appear to have a critical role by regulating binding of the polymerase on the RNA template [19,20], and miR-122 also plays a role in HCV replication [14]. NS5B polymerase lacks proofreading activity and therefore HCV has high mutation rates (as is the case for most RNA viruses).

Assembly and release

Assembly and release of newly formed HCV particles are two events intimately linked to lipid metabolism. The first event in HCV assembly is the targeting of the core protein from the ER membrane, where it is translated, to particular cytoplasmic organelles called lipid droplets [21] (believed to be the platform of HCV assembly). The HCV RNA is relocated from the membranous web to lipid droplets in a mechanism that is dependent on the presence of NS5A on core coated-lipid droplets [22]. Trafficking of the core protein and NS5A seems to be partly regulated by one host protein, the diacylglycerol O-acyltransferase 1 (DGAT1) [23]. Other host proteins involved in lipid droplet morphogenesis, such as tail-interacting protein of 47 kDa (TIP47) (a lipid droplet-associated protein) [24] or seipin (involved in lipid droplet maturation) [25], seem to also play a role in assembly. Capsids subsequently migrate in the ER lumen and the viral envelope is acquired by budding of the ER membrane, where HCV glycoproteins E1 and E2 are anchored at the proximity of the assembly site. This final step of assembly is orchestrated by NS2 [26]. Finally, the nascent HCV particles undergo maturation through the VLDL secretory pathway during which they are associated with lipoproteins before being released by exocytosis as LVPs [27].

> *Key points*
>
> - The hepatitis C virus particle is a spherical (ø ~40–80 nm), enveloped virus (envelope contains viral glycoproteins E1 and E2), with a single-strand positive-sense RNA genome.
> - The virus has an icosahedral capsid structure composed of core protein and circulates as lipo-viro-particles within the blood.
> - The life cycle of HCV targets hepatocytes and consists of seven steps: attachment, entry, uncoating, RNA translation and polyprotein maturation, RNA replication, particle assembly on lipid droplets, and release.

References

1   Bradley DW, McCaustland KA, Cook EH, Schable CA, Ebert JW, Maynard JE. Posttransfusion non-A, non-B hepatitis in chimpanzees. Physicochemical evidence that the tubule-forming agent is a small, enveloped virus. *Gastroenterology*. 1985;88:773–779.

2   Gastaminza P, Dryden KA, Boyd B, et al. Ultrastructural and biophysical characterization of hepatitis C virus particles produced in cell culture. *J Virol*. 2010;84:10999–11009.

3   Choo QL, Richman KH, Han JH, et al. Genetic organization and diversity of the hepatitis C virus. *Proc Natl Acad Sci U S A*. 1991;88:2451–2455.

4   Xu Z, Choi J, Yen TS, et al. Synthesis of a novel hepatitis C virus protein by ribosomal frameshift. *EMBO J*. 2001;20:3840–3848.

5   Komurian-Pradel F, Rajoharison A, Berland JL, et al. Antigenic relevance of F protein in chronic hepatitis C virus infection. *Hepatology*. 2004;40:900–909.

6   Fraser CS, Doudna JA. Structural and mechanistic insights into hepatitis C viral translation initiation. *Nat Rev Microbiol*. 2007;5:29–38.

7   Bai Y, Zhou K, Doudna JA. Hepatitis C virus 3′UTR regulates viral translation through direct interactions with the host translation machinery. *Nucleic Acids Res*. 2013;41:7861–7874.

8   Andre P, Komurian-Pradel F, Deforges S, et al. Characterization of low- and very-low-density hepatitis C virus RNA-containing particles. *J Virol*. 2002;76:6919–6928.

9   Agnello V, Abel G, Elfahal M, Knight GB, Zhang QX. Hepatitis C virus and other flaviviridae viruses enter cells via low density lipoprotein receptor. *Proc Natl Acad Sci U S A*. 1999;96:12766–12771.

10 Scarselli E, Ansuini H, Cerino R, et al. The human scavenger receptor class B type I is a novel candidate receptor for the hepatitis C virus. *EMBO J*. 2002;21:5017–5025.

11 Bartosch B, Verney G, Dreux M, et al, An interplay between hypervariable region 1 of the hepatitis C virus E2 glycoprotein, the scavenger receptor BI, and high-density lipoprotein promotes both enhancement of infection and protection against neutralizing antibodies. *J Virol*. 2005;79:8217–8229.

12 Farquhar MJ, Hu K, Harris HJ, et al. Hepatitis C virus induces CD81 and claudin-1 endocytosis. *J Virol*. 2012;86:4305–4316.

13 Izumi RE, Das S, Barat B, Raychaudhuri S, Dasgupta A. A peptide from autoantigen La blocks poliovirus and hepatitis C virus cap-independent translation and reveals a single tyrosine critical for La RNA binding and translation stimulation. *J Virol*. 2004;78:3763–3776.

14 Jopling CL, Yi M, Lancaster AM, Lemon SM, Sarnow P. Modulation of hepatitis C virus RNA abundance by a liver-specific MicroRNA. *Science*. 2005;309:1577–1581.

15 Roberts AP, Lewis AP, Jopling CL. miR-122 activates hepatitis C virus translation by a specialized mechanism requiring particular RNA components. *Nucleic Acids Res.* 2011;39:7716–7729.

16 Ray U, Das S. Interplay between NS3 protease and human La protein regulates translation-replication switch of Hepatitis C virus. *Sci Rep.* 2011;1:1.

17 She Y, Liao Q, Chen X, Ye L, Wu Z. Hepatitis C virus (HCV) NS2 protein up-regulates HCV IRES-dependent translation and down-regulates NS5B RdRp activity. *Arch Virol.* 2008;153:1991–1997.

18 Egger D, Wölk B, Gosert R, et al. Expression of hepatitis C virus proteins induces distinct membrane alterations including a candidate viral replication complex. *J Virol.* 2002;76:5974–5984.

19 Watashi K, Ishii N, Hijikata M, et al. Cyclophilin B is a functional regulator of hepatitis C virus RNA polymerase. *Mol Cell.* 2005;19:111–122.

20 Kaul A, Stauffer S, Berger C, et al. Essential role of cyclophilin A for hepatitis C virus replication and virus production and possible link to polyprotein cleavage kinetics. *PLoS Pathog.* 2009;5:e1000546.

21 McLauchlan J, Lemberg MK, Hope G, Martoglio B. Intramembrane proteolysis promotes trafficking of hepatitis C virus core protein to lipid droplets. *EMBO J.* 2002;21:3980–3988.

22 Masaki T, Suzuki R, Murakami K, et al. Interaction of hepatitis C virus nonstructural protein 5A with core protein is critical for the production of infectious virus particles. *J Virol.* 2008;82:7964–7976.

23 Herker E, Harris C, Hernandez C, et al. Efficient hepatitis C virus particle formation requires diacylglycerol acyltransferase-1. *Nat Med.* 2010;16:1295–1298.

24 Vogt DA, Camus G, Herker E, et al. Lipid droplet-binding protein TIP47 regulates hepatitis C Virus RNA replication through interaction with the viral NS5A protein. *PLoS Pathog.* 2013;9:e1003302.

25 Clément S, Fauvelle C, Branche E, et al. Role of seipin in lipid droplet morphology and hepatitis C virus life cycle. *J Gen Virol.* 2013;94(Pt 10):2208–2214.

26 Popescu CI, Callens N, Trinel D, et al. NS2 protein of hepatitis C virus interacts with structural and non-structural proteins towards virus assembly. *PLoS Pathog.* 2011;7:e1001278.

27 Gastaminza P, Kapadia SB, Chisari FV. Differential biophysical properties of infectious intracellular and secreted hepatitis C virus particles. *J Virol.* 2006;80:11074–11081.

Chapter 3

Clinical features

Hepatitis C virus (HCV) infection is generally paucisymptomatic, except during the later stages of disease when complications of chronic HCV infection such as liver decompensation and hepatocellular carcinoma (HCC) occur. In this chapter we review the clinical features associated with acute and chronic HCV infection, including extrahepatic manifestations, and discuss factors associated with disease progression.

Acute and chronic HCV infection

Following infection with HCV, the acute phase of HCV infection is generally asymptomatic or rather unrecognized by the patient or physician. When symptoms are present they are mild and generally aspecific but may include fatigue, flu-like symptoms, dyspepsia, or jaundice (during a period of 2–12 weeks following infection). Serologically, HCV RNA will only be detectable 1–3 weeks after HCV infection, whereas seroconversion may take place 4–10 weeks after exposure [1]. In practice, the first sign of liver injury will be rising alanine aminotransferase (ALT) levels 4–12 weeks after infection. Thus, even in the absence of symptoms, elevated serum ALT levels, especially in at-risk individuals (intravenous drug users, parenteral exposure to HCV), should trigger further testing for HCV infection. Spontaneous resolution of the infection generally occurs within 3 months after infection; however, the majority of patients will progress toward chronic infection if untreated.

Chronic HCV infection is defined as persistence of detectable HCV RNA levels for more than 6 months after initial infection. The probability

© Springer International Publishing Switzerland 2016
N. Goossens et al. (eds.), *Handbook of Hepatitis C*,
DOI 10.1007/978-3-319-28053-0_3

of progressing to chronic HCV after an acute infection has been reported to be 55–85%, although this is likely an underestimate and most patients probably progress to chronic disease if asymptomatic acute infections are taken into account [2,3]. Factors linked to an increased risk of developing chronic HCV include host *IFNL3* polymorphisms, human immunodeficiency virus (HIV) co-infection, and asymptomatic acute HCV infection [4].

Natural history of chronic HCV infection

Once chronic HCV infection is established, the natural history is remarkably variable and influenced by a number of cofactors. In general, the progression to cirrhosis will take decades. In a large systematic review of prognostic studies Thein et al [5] found the prevalence of cirrhosis at 20 years after infection to be 16% (Figure 3.1). Alternatively, in a homogeneous cohort of young women infected by anti-D immunoglobulin in Germany, fibrosis progression rates were slower, with 15% of patients being cirrhotic at a 35-year follow-up [6].

Hepatic decompensation

The risk of hepatic decompensation and HCC development increases significantly after cirrhosis has occurred. Hepatic decompensation is characterized by the development of jaundice, ascites, variceal bleeding,

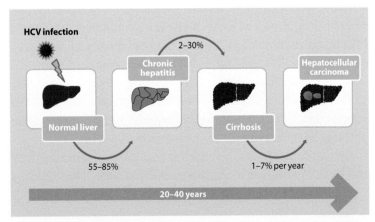

Figure 3.1 The natural history of hepatitis C virus infection [5–12]. This figure was produced using Servier Medical Art, available from www.servier.com/Powerpoint-image-bank.

and encephalopathy. In a retrospective study of patients with HCV and compensated cirrhosis, 18% of patients developed liver decompensation at 5-years of follow-up, whereas 7% developed HCC [7]. Importantly, in an analysis of the Hepatitis C Antiviral Long-term Treatment against Cirrhosis (HALT-C) Trial (NCT00006164), after development of a Child-Turcotte-Pugh score ≥7 the rate of subsequent events increased to 12.9% per year, including a death rate of 10% per year, underlining the increased morbidity and mortality linked to even moderate signs of liver decompensation [8].

Hepatocellular carcinoma

HCV infection is the leading etiology of HCC in developed countries; 50–60% of patients with HCC in the US are infected with HCV [9]. HCC rarely develops in livers with less fibrosis, although the risk of HCC increases as liver fibrosis progresses. The annual incidence of HCC in patients with established cirrhosis is 1–7% per year [10]. Crucially, despite sustained virological response (SVR) after antiviral therapy, the risk of HCC is reduced but not eliminated, especially in patients with advanced fibrosis [11].

Overall survival

As expected, overall survival is decreased in patients with chronic HCV infection, driven in part by increased liver-related deaths [12]. In the US, HCV is responsible for 4.58 deaths per 100,000 persons per year [12]. Additionally, depending on concomitant risk factors, it is becoming increasingly clear that mortality from extrahepatic causes, including renal and cardiovascular mortality, is also increased in patients with HCV (independent of the stage of fibrosis) [13]. Thus, treating patients with HCV infection may reduce the occurrence of liver-related and extrahepatic outcomes.

Clinical manifestations

Clinical manifestations of HCV infection are variable, but can be broadly classified into hepatic and extrahepatic manifestations.

Hepatic manifestations

Most patients in the early stages of chronic HCV infection are asymptomatic or have only mild non-specific symptoms such as fatigue, nausea, anorexia, weight loss, or arthralgia. Following the development of cirrhosis, patients may develop liver decompensation. In a review by Planas et al [14] of 200 cases of decompensated HCV cirrhosis, the most common sign of first hepatic decompensation in chronic HCV infection was ascites (48%), followed by variceal bleeding (32.5%), bacterial infection (14.5%), and hepatic encephalopathy (5%). During a mean follow-up of 34 months, 16.5% of patients developed HCC and death occurred in 42.5%, highlighting the high morbidity and mortality of patients with HCV presenting with hepatic decompensation [14]. Importantly, clinical manifestations of HCV cirrhosis are clinically indistinguishable from other etiologies of liver disease.

Extrahepatic manifestations

Extrahepatic manifestations of chronic HCV infection are likely multifactorial, may be severe, and can lead to greater morbidity in some cases (Figure 3.2) [15].

Hematologic disorders

Specific hematologic disorders, including essential mixed cryoglobulinemia and B cell non-Hodgkin lymphoma, have been linked to chronic HCV infection. Essential mixed cryoglobulinemia (also called type II mixed cryoglobulinemia, monoclonal IgM, and polyclonal IgG) is found in 19–50% of patients with chronic HCV, generally at low titers and clinically asymptomatic. However, in 4–10% of all patients with HCV mixed cryoglobulinemia clinically manifests, most commonly with weakness, arthralgia, and purpura (the so-called Meltzer triad). Patients may develop leukocytoclastic vasculitis that will present clinically as palpable purpura and petechiae, generally involving the lower extremities. More serious manifestations of cryoglobulinemia include neurologic disease (peripheral neuropathy) and renal disease (usually membranoproliferative glomerulonephritis). Management of mixed cryoglobulinemia in the setting of HCV infection is complex and may require a combination of

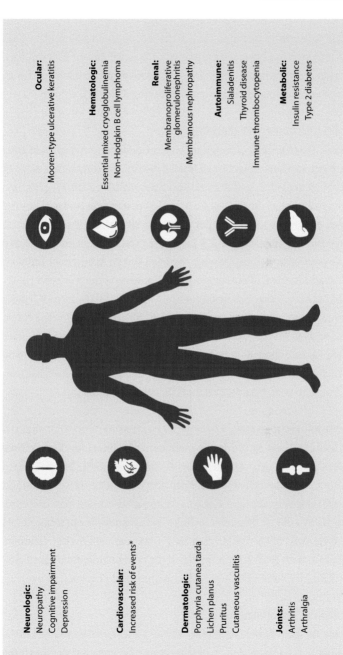

Neurologic:
Neuropathy
Cognitive impairment
Depression

Cardiovascular:
Increased risk of events*

Dermatologic:
Porphyria cutanea tarda
Lichen planus
Pruritus
Cutaneous vasculitis

Joints:
Arthritis
Arthralgia

Ocular:
Mooren-type ulcerative keratitis

Hematologic:
Essential mixed cryoglobulinemia
Non-Hodgkin B cell lymphoma

Renal:
Membranoproliferative
glomerulonephritis
Membranous nephropathy

Autoimmune:
Sialadenitis
Thyroid disease
Immune thrombocytopenia

Metabolic:
Insulin resistance
Type 2 diabetes

Figure 3.2 Extrahepatic manifestations of hepatitis C virus infection by organ. Information adapted from Negro et al [15]. * Denotes further research is required.

immunosuppressive therapy and HCV therapy, depending on severity [16]. HCV infection has been associated with the development of B cell non-Hodgkin lymphoma [17, 18]. Viral eradication may be associated with lower risk of lymphoma in patients achieving SVR [19].

Insulin resistance and diabetes

Clinical, experimental, and epidemiological evidence converge to suggest that there is a link between HCV and insulin resistance that may, in susceptible patients, lead to type 2 diabetes mellitus (T2DM) [20]. In a large systematic review by White et al [21] of over 300,000 patients the pooled estimate of T2DM in patients with HCV was an adjusted odds ratio (OR) of approximately 1.7. Insulin resistance may not only lead to cardiovascular complications, but has been shown to be associated with worsened response to antiviral therapy (at least with interferon [IFN]-based regimens) and increased rates of HCC [22,23]. Curing HCV with antiviral therapy has been shown to result in reduction of insulin resistance; however, virological non-responders did not demonstrate this benefit [24]. Danoprevir, a HCV non-structural protein (NS)3/4A protease inhibitor, showed similar effects in the improvement of insulin sensitivity in a Phase Ib trial in patients with HCV genotype 1 [25].

Dermatologic disease

The sporadic form of porphyria cutanea tarda (PCT) has been shown to have a strong association with HCV infection [26]. The two main clinical manifestations of PCT are hepatic (inflammation, steatosis, and fibrosis) and dermatologic disease (photosensitivity and skin fragility). Management of PCT generally includes avoidance of precipitating factors and treatment of the underlying HCV infection. Other skin disorders associated with HCV infection include the cryoglobulinemia-associated vasculitis, as described above, lichen planus, and pruritus.

Neurologic manifestations

The involvement of the peripheral nervous system is closely linked to the presence of essential mixed cryoglobulinemia. Pathological findings often show ischemic nerve changes, a consequence of small vessel vasculitis, leading to a symmetrical sensory or sensorimotor axonal-type polyneuropathy with sensory loss and weakness in distal regions of limbs [27]. Alternatively, clinical presentation may include mononeuropathies or mononeuritis multiplex, with usual sparing of cranial nerves.

Although involvement of the peripheral nervous system during HCV infection is well documented, there is also an association with central nervous system disorders. Patients with HCV have a reduced quality of life due to a decrease in physical and mental health and more than 50% report fatigue [28]. In addition, regardless of the severity of the liver disease, a mild deficiency in attention and memory has also been reported [29]. Regardless of pre-existing psychiatric disorders, patients with HCV infection are more likely to have comorbid neuropsychiatric symptoms, such as drug and alcohol abuse, major depression, bipolar disorder, and schizophrenia [30].

Other extrahepatic manifestations

There are a number of other extrahepatic manifestations of HCV, including auto-immune manifestations (thyroid disease, sialadenitis, and immune thrombocytopenia) and ophthalmological disease (especially Mooren-type peripheral ulcerative keratitis). In addition, despite a generally 'cardioprotective' serum lipid profile with low total cholesterol, low-density lipoprotein, and triglycerides, and high high-density lipoprotein compared to uninfected individuals [31], several retrospective and prospective studies have suggested an increased cardiovascular risk in HCV-positive individuals [15]. However, it remains unclear whether HCV infection is independently linked to increased cardiovascular outcomes or whether its association with other cardiovascular risk factors, such as diabetes, drives this increase.

Prognosis and factors affecting disease progression

There is a remarkable variability in HCV disease progression between individuals; this is due to a number of well characterized viral factors and host factors, as detailed in the following sections.

Viral factors associated with disease progression

HCV RNA titers have not been associated with prognosis and overall disease progression, although viral genotype seems to play a prognostic role. HCV genotype 3 has been associated with increased fibrosis progression rates [32] and increased rates of HCC [11,33,34]. In addition, genotype 3 has also been associated with reduced response rates to non-IFN based antiviral therapy [33].

Host factors associated with disease progression

One of the main factors associated with disease progression is the amount of intrahepatic inflammation linked to HCV infection. This was demonstrated in a meta-analysis of individual data of 3068 patients that showed that histological activity was significantly associated with fibrosis stage (adjusted OR greater than 5) [35].

Male sex is associated with accelerated fibrosis progression rates and higher HCC incidence, although this observation may be (at least in part) linked to hormonal effects as menopause is associated with a significant increase in fibrosis progression in women [35,36]. Recent reports have underlined the key role played by host genetic polymorphisms. In 590 patients with an estimated date of infection and a subsequent liver biopsy, variations in *TULP1*, *MERTK,* and *PNPLA3* genes and the major histocompatibility complex (MHC) region were associated with accelerated fibrosis progression rates [37]. Age at infection also seems to play a role, as patients infected at a younger age seem to have lower rates of disease progression.

A number of key modifiable host factors are tightly linked to HCV disease progression and prognosis. Crucially, alcohol use should be kept to a minimum by all patients with chronic HCV infection as alcohol abuse has been associated with accelerated disease progression and worse outcomes [38]. By contrast, a number of concordant studies seem to suggest a hepatoprotective role of coffee [39,40]. With the current worldwide epidemic of obesity and features of the metabolic syndrome, it is particularly worrying that steatosis, diabetes, and insulin resistance are all linked to increased progression and increased rates of HCC in patients with HCV [13].

The role of hepatitis B co-infection on disease progression is still being elucidated, although it is clear that HIV and HCV co-infection leads to increased fibrosis progression rates and this negative effect may not be completely reversible even with active antiretroviral therapy [41]. Similarly, if untreated prior to liver transplantation, re-infection of the graft after transplantation is universal and fibrosis progression is markedly increased compared to non-transplanted controls [42].

Conclusion

Hepatitis C is a protean and clinically inconspicuous disease, therefore the threshold for testing individuals should be low, especially in at-risk individuals. If unidentified and left untreated, complications of HCV may arise within years to decades, depending on a number of host and viral factors.

Key points

- HCV infection is generally paucisymptomatic in the early stages of infection; however, complications of chronic HCV infection occur during the later stages of disease (liver decompensation and HCC).
- Symptoms, when present, are mild and generally aspecific but may include fatigue, flu-like symptoms, dyspepsia, or jaundice.
- Even in the absence of symptoms, elevated serum ALT levels (especially in at-risk individuals) should trigger further testing for HCV infection.
- A majority of patients will progress toward chronic HCV infection if untreated.
- Non-modifiable factors affecting disease progression include hepatitis C virus genotype (genotype 3 causing the most rapid progression), intrahepatic inflammation, male sex, older age at infection, genetic polymorphisms, and HIV co-infection.
- Modifiable factors affecting disease progression include alcohol consumption and metabolic syndrome.

- Clinical manifestations are broadly divided into hepatic manifestations (eg, cirrhosis and liver decompensation) and extrahepatic manifestations (including hematologic disorders, insulin resistance and diabetes, dermatologic disease, neurologic manifestations, auto-immune manifestations, and ophthalmological disease).

References

1   Santantonio T, Wiegand J, Gerlach JT. Acute hepatitis C: current status and remaining challenges. *J Hepatol*. 2008;49:625–633.

2   Gerlach JT, Diepolder HM, Zachoval R, et al. Acute hepatitis C: high rate of both spontaneous and treatment-induced viral clearance. *Gastroenterology*. 2003;125:80–88.

3   Seeff LB. Natural history of chronic hepatitis C. *Hepatology*. 2002;36 (Suppl 1):S35–46.

4   Negro F. Hepatitis C Virus Epidemiology, Pathogenesis, Diagnosis, and Natural History. In: Zeuzem S, Afdhal NH, editors. *inPractice Hepatology*. 2015.

5   Thein HH, Yi Q, Dore GJ, Krahn MD. Estimation of stage-specific fibrosis progression rates in chronic hepatitis C virus infection: a meta-analysis and meta-regression. *Hepatology*. 2008;48:418–431.

6   Wiese M, Fischer J, Löbermann M, et al. Evaluation of liver disease progression in the German hepatitis C virus (1b)-contaminated anti-D cohort at 35 years after infection. *Hepatology*. 2014;59:49–57.

7   Fattovich G, Giustina G, Degos F, et al. Morbidity and mortality in compensated cirrhosis type C: a retrospective follow-up study of 384 patients. *Gastroenterology*. 1997;112:463–472.

8   Dienstag JL, Ghany MG, Morgan TR, et al. A prospective study of the rate of progression in compensated, histologically advanced chronic hepatitis C. *Hepatology*. 2011;54:396–405.

9   El-Serag HB. Epidemiology of viral hepatitis and hepatocellular carcinoma. *Gastroenterology*. 2012;142:1264–1273.

10 Hoshida Y, Fuchs BC, Bardeesy N, Baumert TF, Chung RT. Pathogenesis and prevention of hepatitis C virus-induced hepatocellular carcinoma. *J Hepatol*. 2014;61 (Suppl 1):S79–90.

11 van der Meer AJ, Veldt BJ, Feld JJ, et al. Association between sustained virological response and all-cause mortality among patients with chronic hepatitis C and advanced hepatic fibrosis. *JAMA*. 2012;308:2584–2593.

12 Ly KN, Xing J, Klevens RM, Jiles RB, Ward JW, Holmberg SD. The increasing burden of mortality from viral hepatitis in the United States between 1999 and 2007. *Ann Intern Med*. 2012;156:271–278.

13 Negro F. Facts and fictions of HCV and comorbidities: steatosis, diabetes mellitus, and cardiovascular diseases. *J Hepatol*. 2014;61 (Suppl 1):S69–78.

14 Planas R, Ballesté B, Alvarez MA, et al. Natural history of decompensated hepatitis C virus-related cirrhosis. A study of 200 patients. *J Hepatol*. 2004;40:823–830.

15 Negro F, Forton D, Craxì A, Sulkowski MS, Feld JJ, Manns MP. Extrahepatic Morbidity and Mortality of Chronic Hepatitis C. *Gastroenterology*. 2015;149:1345–1360.

16 Dammacco F, Sansonno D. Therapy for hepatitis C virus-related cryoglobulinemic vasculitis. *N Eng J Med*. 2013;369:1035–1045.

17 Giordano TP, Henderson L, Landgren O, et al. Risk of non-Hodgkin lymphoma and lymphoproliferative precursor diseases in US veterans with hepatitis C virus. *JAMA*. 2007;297:2010–2017.

18 Gisbert JP, García-Buey L, Pajares JM, Moreno-Otero R. Prevalence of hepatitis C virus infection in B-cell non-Hodgkin's lymphoma: systematic review and meta-analysis. *Gastroenterology*. 2003;125:1723–1732.

19 Kawamura Y, Ikeda K, Arase Y, et al. Viral elimination reduces incidence of malignant lymphoma in patients with hepatitis C. *Am J Med*. 2007;120:1034–1041.

20 Goossens N, Negro F. Insulin Resistance, non-alcoholic fatty liver disease and hepatitis C virus infection. *Rev Recent Clin Trials*. 2014;9:204–209.

21 White DL, Ratziu V, El-Serag HB. Hepatitis C infection and risk of diabetes: a systematic review and meta-analysis. *J Hepatol*. 2008;49:831–844.

22 Romero-Gómez M, Fernández-Rodríguez CM, Andrade RJ, et al. Effect of sustained virological response to treatment on the incidence of abnormal glucose values in chronic hepatitis C. *J Hepatol*. 2008;48:721–727.

23 El-Serag HB, Hampel H, Javadi F. The association between diabetes and hepatocellular carcinoma: a systematic review of epidemiologic evidence. *Clin Gastroenterol Hepatol*. 2006;4:369–380.

24 Kawaguchi T, Ide T, Taniguchi E, et al. Clearance of HCV improves insulin resistance, beta-cell function, and hepatic expression of insulin receptor substrate 1 and 2. *Am J Gastroenterol*. 2007;102:570–576.

25 Moucari R, Forestier N, Larrey D, et al. Danoprevir, an HCV NS3/4A protease inhibitor, improves insulin sensitivity in patients with genotype 1 chronic hepatitis C. *Gut*. 2010;59:1694–1698.

26 Gisbert JP, García-Buey L, Pajares JM, Moreno-Otero R. Prevalence of hepatitis C virus infection in porphyria cutanea tarda: systematic review and meta-analysis. *J Hepatol*. 2003;39:620–627.

27 Gemignani F, Brindani F, Alfieri S, et al. Clinical spectrum of cryoglobulinaemic neuropathy. *J Neuro Neurosurg Psychiatry*. 2005;76:1410–1414.

28 Poynard T, Cacoub P, Ratziu, et al. Fatigue in patients with chronic hepatitis C. *J Viral Hepat*. 2002;9:295–303.

29 Forton DM, Thomas HC, Murphy CA, et al. Hepatitis C and cognitive impairment in a cohort of patients with mild liver disease. *Hepatology*. 2002;35:433–439.

30 Schaefer M, Capuron L, Friebe A, et al. Hepatitis C infection, antiviral treatment and mental health: a European expert consensus statement. *J Hepatol*. 2012;57:1379–1390.

31 Dai CY, Chuang WL, Ho CK, et al. Associations between hepatitis C viremia and low serum triglyceride and cholesterol levels: a community-based study. *J Hepatol*. 2008;49:9–16.

32 Bochud PY, Cai T, Overbeck K, et al. Genotype 3 is associated with accelerated fibrosis progression in chronic hepatitis C. *J Hepatol*. 2009;51:655–666.

33 Goossens N, Negro F. Is genotype 3 of the hepatitis C virus the new villain? *Hepatology*. 2014;59:2403–2412.

34 Nkontchou G, Ziol M, Aout M, et al. HCV genotype 3 is associated with a higher hepatocellular carcinoma incidence in patients with ongoing viral C cirrhosis. *J Viral Hepatitis*. 2011;18:e516–522.

35 Leandro G, Mangia A, Hui J, et al. Relationship between steatosis, inflammation, and fibrosis in chronic hepatitis C: a meta-analysis of individual patient data. *Gastroenterology*. 2006;130:1636–1642.

36 Di Martino V, Lebray P, Myers RP, et al. Progression of liver fibrosis in women infected with hepatitis C: long-term benefit of estrogen exposure. *Hepatology*. 2004;40:1426–1433.

37 Rüeger S, Bochud PY, Dufour JF, et al. Impact of common risk factors of fibrosis progression in chronic hepatitis C. *Gut*. 2015;64:1605–1615.

38 Wiley TE, McCarthy M, Breidi L, McCarthy M, Layden TJ. Impact of alcohol on the histological and clinical progression of hepatitis C infection. *Hepatology*. 1998;28:805–809.

39 Freedman ND, Everhart JE, Lindsay KL, et al. Coffee intake is associated with lower rates of liver disease progression in chronic hepatitis C. *Hepatology*. 2009;50:1360–1369.

40   Cardin R, Piciocchi M, Martines D, Scribano L, Petracco M, Farinati F. Effects of coffee consumption in chronic hepatitis C: a randomized controlled trial. *Dig Liver Dis*. 2013;45:499–504.

41   Thein HH, Yi Q, Dore GJ, Krahn MD. Natural history of hepatitis C virus infection in HIV-infected individuals and the impact of HIV in the era of highly active antiretroviral therapy: a meta-analysis. *AIDS*. 2008;22:1979–1991.

42   Germani G, Tsochatzis E, Papastergiou V, Burroughs AK. HCV in liver transplantation. *Semin Immunopathol*. 2013;35:101–110.

Chapter 4

Pathophysiology

Immune response

In hepatitis C virus (HCV) infection liver damage is not due to direct effects of the virus; the immune response plays a primordial role in the pathophysiology of the disease.

Innate immunity

The first line of defense of the body against pathogens is the non-specific innate immune response. One main characteristic of the innate immune response is the capacity of the infected cell to recognize pathogen components (known as pathogen-associated molecular patterns [PAMPs]) as foreign. Cellular receptors, called pattern recognition receptors (PRRs), sense PAMPs and binding of these viral constituents with PRRs activate a cascade of reactions that leads to the synthesis of cytokines (such as type I interferon [IFN]). Secreted cytokines function locally by binding receptors on neighboring cells, which consequently activates the janus kinase/signal transducer and activator of transcription (Jak/STAT) signaling pathway, leading to the transcription of hundreds of genes (interferon stimulated genes, [ISGs]), and therefore inducing an antiviral state.

In HCV infection, hepatocytes sense particular HCV RNA genome structures (double-stranded RNA [dsRNA] or single-stranded RNA [ssRNA] with a $5'$-triphosphate) that are unusual nucleic acids to be found in cells. Detection of these nucleic acids is via two distinct PRRs; Toll-like receptor-3 (TLR-3) and retinoic acid-inducible gene-I (RIG-I) [1]. HCV

© Springer International Publishing Switzerland 2016
N. Goossens et al. (eds.), *Handbook of Hepatitis C*,
DOI 10.1007/978-3-319-28053-0_4

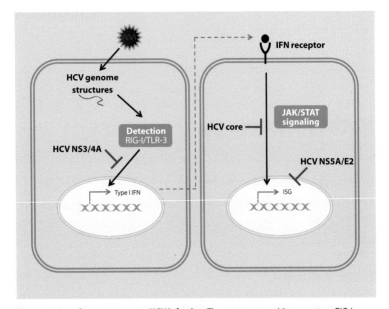

Figure 4.1 Interferon response to HCV infection. The pattern recognition receptors, RIG-I and TLR-3, in infected hepatocytes sense particular HCV RNA genome structures, activating the transcription of type I interferon (type I IFN), which binds to neighboring cells and in turn leads to the transcription of ISGs, via the activation of the Jak/STAT pathway. HCV interferes with interferon response at several levels: the protease NS3/4A can cleave TRIF and IPS-1 involved in the RIG-I/TLR-3 signaling pathway; HCV core protein can block Jak/STAT signaling; and NS5A and E2 can inhibit the antiviral function of some ISGs. E, envelope; HCV, hepatitis C virus; IFN, interferon; JAK, Janus kinase; NS, non-structural; RIG-I, retinoic acid-inducible gene 1; TLR-3, Toll-like receptor 3. This figure was produced using Servier Medical Art, available from www.servier.com/Powerpoint-image-bank.

has evolved strategies to counteract the IFN response (Figure 4.1). The viral protease NS3/4A not only acts during the maturation of the HCV polyprotein but also cleaves two molecules, Toll/interleukin-1 receptor-domain-containing adapter-inducing IFN-β (TRIF) [2] and IFN-β promoter stimulator 1 (IPS-1) [3], involved in the RIG-I/TLR-3 signaling pathway. HCV core protein interferes with innate immune responses by blocking Jak/STAT signaling [4,5]. Some other HCV proteins, such as non-structural protein (NS)5A [6,7] and envelope protein (E)2 [8], can also directly interfere with ISGs, thereby inhibiting their antiviral function.

The innate immune system, in addition to the recognition of foreign components by PRRs, also consists of specific cells, such as dendritic cells (DCs) and natural killer (NK) cells, which are key actors in the immune response to viral infection. Cytokines produced by infected cells bind to DCs, which in turn produce more cytokines, leading to an amplification of the immune response. DCs also play a key role in priming the adaptive immune response by acting as antigen-presenting cells. NK cells have the ability to recognize and kill infected cells. NK cells recognize cells that have down-regulated major histocompatibility complex (MHC) class I molecules on their cell surface (an attempt to evade host immune responses), as well as other signals associated with viral infection (eg, MHC class I chain-related molecules). NK cells possess secretory lysosomes within their cytoplasms, where cytotoxic molecules are stored, ready for release into infected cells via tightly regulated and ordered exocytosis [9].

In HCV infection both cell types play an important role in the host immune response and their impairment may, in part, explain the establishment of chronic infection. In chronic HCV infection, NK cells are present in the liver and are activated, but they fail to clear the virus. It has been shown that NK cells from patients infected with HCV express a high level of CD94/NKG2A inhibitory receptors, which alter their activation (and the activation of DCs) [10]. In addition, the HCV envelope protein, E2, binds to CD81 (highly expressed on NK cells) to inhibit non-MHC-restricted cytotoxicity and the production of IFN-γ, thus altering their functions [11]. The maturation and differentiation of plasmacytoid (pDCs) and conventional (cDCs) DCs are impaired in patients with chronic HCV infection. In the case of pDCs, HCV proteins (such as core protein and NS3) appear to reduce IFN-α production and induce pDC apoptosis either directly or via a monocyte-mediated mechanism [12,13]. Similarly, cDCs appear to display alteration in cytokine production [14], which may lead to delayed HCV-specific T cell priming, although this theory remains controversial and further research is required.

Adaptive immune responses

In general, the adaptive immune response takes place upon activation by innate immune actors. The main cells involved in the adaptive response are T and B lymphocytes, which allow a highly specific defense against infectious agents. Two types of T lymphocyte, CD4+ (helper) and CD8+

(cytotoxic) T cells, display different functions, both of which are extremely important in immune defense. Following activation by antigen presenting cells, CD4+ T cells proliferate and secrete soluble molecules, such as interleukin (IL)-2, which stimulate T and B cell proliferation as well as activate macrophages. Activated CD8+ T cells acquire the ability to kill infected cells by producing molecules such as perforin or granzyme. When B lymphocytes are activated they differentiate into effector B cells and produce specific antibodies against viral antigens to neutralize them.

HCV can induce an adaptive immune response (Figure 4.2A); however, it is particularly delayed, as HCV-specific T cells and antibodies are usually only detectable 5–9 weeks and 8–20 weeks after infection, respectively [15,16]. Additionally, even though most patients produce antibodies against HCV epitopes, the majority of these antibodies do not display neutralizing activity and fail to clear the virus. It is worth noting that an early production of neutralizing antibodies has been correlated with HCV clearance [17], but so far their real implication in this process has not been fully established and it has been observed that HCV can be cleared in absence of humoral response (eg, in patients with hypogammaglobulinemia) [18]. HCV appears to induce the production of antibodies and the proliferation of B cells that are not specific for HCV [19], which can lead in some cases to the development of type II mixed cryoglobulinemia or non-Hodgkin lymphoma [20].

Conversely, T cell response is absolutely essential for HCV clearance [15]. Studies in chimpanzees have demonstrated that the depletion of either subset of T cells leads to HCV persistence [21,22]. In addition, a correlation has been established between the presence of HCV-specific CD4+ T cells in the blood of patients during the acute phase of infection and clearance of the virus [23]. However, in most patients, HCV can persist despite the establishment of adaptive immune responses (Figure 4.2B). Several mechanisms have been proposed to explain the failure of these responses:

• the lack of proofreading activity of HCV polymerase can lead to virus escape from neutralizing antibodies as well as from the T cell response [24];

- the presence of specific glycans on the E2 envelope protein protects HCV from neutralization by antibodies [25];
- virions inglobated into particles rich in host-derived lipids, the so-called lipo-viro-particles (LVPs);
- T cell exhaustion, defined by impaired cell functions and proliferation (often observed in patients with HCV);
- HCV-specific CD8+ T cells are characterized by a high expression of inhibitory receptors, such as programmed death–1 (PD-1), which, upon binding to its ligand PD-L1 (expressed on several types of cells in the liver, eg, Kupffer cells, stellate cells, and hepatocytes), promotes T cell apoptosis [26].
  - However, treatment with antibodies targeting PD-1 can only partially restore the function of CD8+ T cells [27], indicating that T cell exhaustion is not only mediated by PD-1 but also by the co-expression of other inhibitory receptors. For instance, 2B4 (CD244), killer cell lectin-like receptor G1 (KLRG1), and CD160 have been shown to be highly expressed by HCV-specific CD8+ T cells [28].
- another hallmark of HCV chronic infection is the proliferation of CD4+CD25+ T regulatory cells, which have the ability to suppress immune responses of other cells [29,30].

Molecular mechanisms of liver injury

HCV almost exclusively infects hepatocytes and thus induces liver injury, including fibrosis, cirrhosis, and hepatocellular carcinoma (HCC).

Microscopic anatomy and histology of the liver

The liver is the largest internal organ in the human body and is divided into four lobes (right, left, caudate, and quadrate lobes). The liver receives blood from two different origins:

- the hepatic artery — brings the oxygen-rich blood to the liver; and
- the hepatic portal vein — brings blood containing nutrients absorbed from the gastrointestinal tract to the liver.

The structural unit of the liver, the hepatic lobule, is a hexagonal structure formed of hepatocytes that are well organized around a central vein

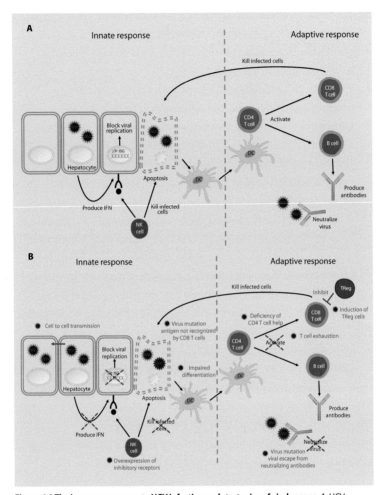

Figure 4.2 The immune response to HCV infection and strategies of viral escape. A, HCV induces the innate immune response (interferon signaling, dendritic cells, and natural killer cell activation), which primes the adaptive immune response (CD4+ [helper] and CD8+ [cytotoxic] T cells and antibody-producing B cells). B, HCV evolves several mechanisms contributing to the failure of immune response and the establishment of chronic infection (see text for more detail). This figure was produced using Servier Medical Art, available from www.servier.com/Powerpoint-image-bank.

(carries deoxygenated blood away from the liver). At each of the corners of the lobule the so-called portal space can be found. This space contains a branch of the hepatic artery, a branch of the hepatic portal vein, and a bile duct. Blood coming from hepatic portal vein and hepatic artery

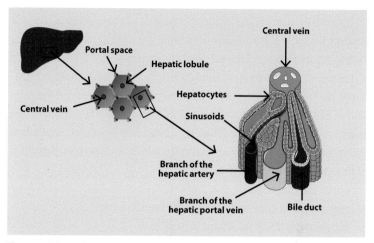

Figure 4.3 Schematic representation of the liver. The hepatic lobule contains hepatocytes organized around a central vein. The portal space found at each of the corners of the lobule contains a branch of the hepatic artery, a branch of the hepatic portal vein, and a bile duct. This figure was produced using Servier Medical Art, available from www.servier.com/Powerpoint-image-bank.

travels through capillaries, called sinusoids, to reach the central vein (Figure 4.3). Histologically, the liver is mainly composed of hepatocytes, but other types of cells are also found, including sinusoidal endothelial cells and Kupffer cells (liver resident macrophages), hepatic stellate cells (HSC) found in spaces of Disse (located between sinusoids and hepatocytes), and resident immune cells (such as lymphocytes).

Fibrogenesis and cirrhosis

Chronic hepatitis C is characterized by the inexorable development of liver fibrosis in response to persistent liver injury, which will eventually progress towards cirrhosis after several decades, following a classical wound-healing process. Cirrhosis, the most advanced stage of fibrosis, is characterized by the loss of the liver architecture caused by the progressive formation of fibrotic septa, which delimit nodules to profoundly modify the lobular structure of the liver. These modifications perturb the blood flow within the parenchyma, leading to loss of hepatocyte function and portal hypertension, the two main clinical consequences of cirrhosis.

Fibrosis is a reversible process; reversion of the amount of fibrotic scarring in cases with established cirrhosis is frequently observed among HCV patients with a sustained virologic response (SVR) [31]. Fibrosis is defined as the abnormal accumulation of extracellular matrix (ECM) due to the imbalance between enhanced synthesis and reduced degradation of ECM proteins. Degradation of ECM proteins is regulated by the matrix metalloproteinases (MMPs), a large family of zinc-dependent endopeptidases. In the liver, several cell populations have been described to be potentially fibrogenic, including:

- portal fibroblasts;
- mesenchymal cells derived from the bone marrow;
- fibroblasts derived from hepatocytes;
- biliary epithelial cells, which may undergo epithelial to mesenchymal transition (EMT); and
- HSCs.

Among the cell types listed above, HSCs have been identified as the primary source of ECM in liver fibrosis. In chronic hepatitis C, the fibrogenic process appears to be mainly the result of viral-induced inflammation; inflammatory cells of the intrahepatic infiltrate secrete cytokines and chemokines that induce the activation of HSCs [32]. Transforming growth factor (TGF)-β seems to be the most profibrotic cytokine. Activated HSCs display several activities, including the synthesis of ECM, the secretion of MMPs and tissue inhibitors of metalloproteinases, contractile and migratory activities, and secretion of proinflammatory chemokines (eliciting an amplification of the process). The direct impact of HCV has been reported in studies investigating the role of core protein and E2 on hepatic fibrogenesis [33,34]. In these studies it was demonstrated that viral proteins may directly induce infected hepatocytes to produce cytokines and reactive oxygen species, in turn activating HSCs without the participation of the inflammatory response [33,34]. This process could explain the fact that some patients develop significant liver fibrosis in a non-inflammatory context.

A very important observation is that the liver fibrosis progression rate is highly variable among patients with HCV; ranging from patients without fibrosis (even after several decades of infection) to patients who rapidly develop cirrhosis. A large study by Rüeger et al [35], conducted in the Swiss Hepatitis C Cohort and replicated in three other cohorts, stressed the role of host and viral factors (such as age at infection, sex, route of infection, HCV genotype 3, and the presence of single nucleotide polymorphisms [SNPs] in *PNPLA3* or in the MHC region) in the progression of liver fibrosis.

Steatosis

Steatosis, also known as fatty liver, is characterized by an accumulation of neutral lipids in the cytoplasm of hepatocytes. Etiologies of steatosis include metabolic syndrome, excess alcohol consumption, host SNPs, toxins, or drugs. In chronic hepatitis C, the reported prevalence of steatosis varies between 40 and 86%, much higher than in the general population (suggesting that HCV may directly cause steatosis) [36]. The direct contribution of HCV in the pathogenesis of steatosis is supported by the fact that it tends to decrease with successful antiviral therapy [37]. A strong association between steatosis and HCV genotype 3 is now well recognized [38].

Several non-exclusive molecular mechanisms have been described to account for HCV-induced steatosis (Figure 4.4). First, lipid neosynthesis appears to be increased via the activation of sterol regulatory element binding protein-1c (SREBP-1c), a transcription factor regulating the expression of enzymes involved in fatty acid biosynthesis [39]. Second, lipid secretion seems to be impaired; the low level of apolipoprotein B (ApoB) and cholesterol frequently observed in patients infected with HCV (especially with genotype 3) with steatosis is an argument in favor of fat retention in the liver. This is further supported by the fact that HCV interferes with microsomal triglyceride transfer protein (MTTP), an enzyme that plays a key role in very-low-density lipoprotein (VLDL) assembly [40,41]. Third, HCV also impairs mitochondrial fatty acid oxidation via the down-regulation of the peroxisome proliferator-activated receptor alpha (PPAR-α) [42–44]. Finally, HCV down-regulates the phosphatase and tensin homolog deleted on chromosome 10 (PTEN), which in turn promotes a reduction of insulin receptor substrate 1 (IRS-1) expression, leading to formation of lipid droplets [45].

HCV needs lipids to achieve most steps of its life cycle, suggesting that HCV interferes with lipid metabolism to favor its own viral particle production. The tight relationship between HCV and lipids is illustrated by the following [46]:

- HCV uses lipoprotein receptors — low-density lipoprotein receptor (LDLR) and scavenger receptor class B type 1 (SR-B1);
- the specific membrane structure (the membranous web) in which replication takes place is highly dependent on the lipid composition;

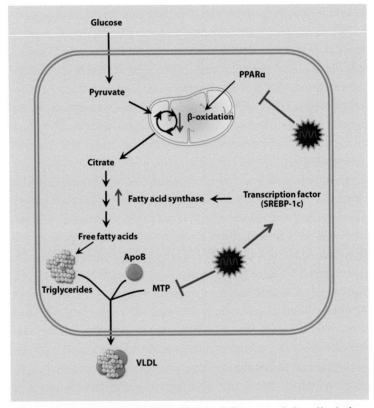

Figure 4.4. The mechanisms by which hepatitis C virus induces steatosis. Several levels of lipid metabolism can be affected by HCV, for example, free fatty acid neosynthesis and lipid β-oxidation or secretion (see text for more detail). ApoB, apolipoprotein B; MTP, microsomal triglyceride transfer protein; PPARα, peroxisome proliferator-activated receptor alpha; SREBP-1c, sterol regulatory element-binding protein 1c; VLDL, very-low-density lipoprotein. This figure was produced using Servier Medical Art, available from www.servier.com/Powerpoint-image-bank.

- particle assembly is believed to occur on lipid droplets; and
- HCV circulates as LVPs.

Pathogenesis of HCV-associated hepatocellular carcinoma

HCC is the fifth most common cancer worldwide and leads to approximately 700,000 deaths per year [47]. Epidemiological studies have indicated that chronic HCV infection is the second most important risk factor for HCC and HCC represents the major cause of death in patients with chronic HCV infection [48]. The pathophysiology of HCC is a complex process and is not fully understood; both indirect and HCV protein-driven direct effects have been documented and implicated in HCC development. The indirect effect of chronic inflammation is certainly an important risk factor for HCC. A large majority of cases of HCC caused by HCV occur in the background of cirrhosis [49]. In this context, repetitive cycles of cell death and regeneration probably contribute to the progression of HCC. Cellular transformation may also be participated by oxidative stress generated from inflammation in chronic HCV infection (Figure 4.5). An interesting feature of HCV is its ability to induce insulin resistance and steatosis, hallmarks of metabolic syndrome, another well recognized risk factor of HCC. Data from a study by Hung et al [50] of 188 patients with different stages of HCV infection suggested that insulin resistance is associated with HCC in chronic hepatitis C infection. A study by Kuske et al [51] of 3390 patients with HCV from the Swiss Hepatitis C Cohort identified diabetes as an independent risk factor of HCC. Steatosis also appears to be an independent risk factor for the development of HCC [52,53], although evidence is limited. Interestingly, multiple studies have pointed out the direct effect of HCV proteins on host gene expression that promote cancer development. More specifically, some pathways involved in tumorigenesis (such as the mitogen-activated protein kinase [MAPK] [54], Wnt/β-catenin [55], and TGF-β [56] pathways) are impaired by the expression of HCV proteins (Figure 4.5). Alternative mechanisms also comprise the activation of oncogenes and/or the inactivation of tumor suppressors by HCV proteins (Figure 4.5), including:

- the transcription of c-Myc (an oncogene contributing to the occurrence of many types of cancers, including HCC, mainly by inducing genetic damage) is increased by NS5A through β-catenin pathway activation [57];
- the function of p53, a tumor suppressor that plays a role in apoptosis, genomic stability, and cell growth and is frequently inactivated in HCC [58], is impaired by HCV infection [59];
- NS5B induces a proteasome-dependent degradation of the Retinoblastoma protein (Rb), another tumor suppressor, subsequently leading to a stimulation of the cell cycle [60]; and
- the HCV core protein induces a decrease of the tumor suppressor, PTEN, which could also contribute to HCC [45].

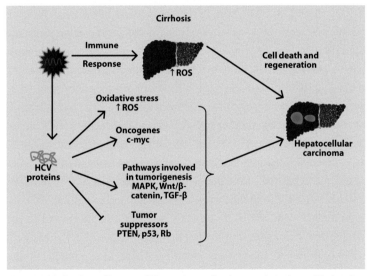

Figure 4.5 Mechanisms of hepatocellular carcinoma development in patients with chronic HCV infection. Nearly all cases of HCC occur in the background of cirrhosis. Oxidative stress due to inflammation may contribute to the development of HCC and HCV proteins can also directly promote HCC by impairing pathways involved in tumorigenesis, thus activating oncogenes and/or inactivating tumor suppressors. HCV, hepatitis C virus; MAPK, mitogen-activated protein kinases; PTEN, phosphatase and tensin homolog deleted on chromosome 10; Rb, Retinoblastoma protein; ROS, reactive oxygen species. This figure was produced using Servier Medical Art, available from www.servier.com/Powerpoint-image-bank.

Key points
- HCV almost exclusively infects hepatocytes and thus induces liver injury, including fibrosis, cirrhosis, and HCC.
- The liver damage seen in HCV infection is due to the immune response rather than direct effects of the virus.
- The innate immune response is crucial in activating an antiviral state and priming the adaptive immune response; however, HCV core protein, NS5A, and E2 interfere with innate immune responses by blocking signaling pathways and inhibiting their antiviral function.
- The adaptive immune response is activated in HCV infection; however, in most patients the virus is not cleared and HCV infection persists.
- Fibrosis (a reversible process) is defined as the abnormal accumulation of ECM due to the imbalance between synthesis and degradation of ECM proteins.
- Cirrhosis, the most advanced stage of fibrosis, is characterized by the loss of liver architecture due to persistent liver injury and wound-healing.
- Steatosis is characterized by an accumulation of neutral lipids in the cytoplasm of hepatocytes and has a prevalence of 40–86% in patients with HCV.
- The pathophysiology of HCC is a complex process and is not fully understood; both indirect and HCV protein-driven direct effects have been documented and implicated.

References

1   Saito T, Owen DM, Jiang F, Marcotrigiano J, Gale M Jr. Innate immunity induced by composition-dependent RIG-I recognition of hepatitis C virus RNA. *Nature*. 2008;454:523–527.

2   Li K, Foy E, Ferreon JC, et al. Immune evasion by hepatitis C virus NS3/4A protease-mediated cleavage of the Toll-like receptor 3 adaptor protein TRIF. *Proc Natl Acad Sci U S A*. 2005;102:2992–2997.

3   Foy E, Li K, Wang C, et al. Regulation of interferon regulatory factor-3 by the hepatitis C virus serine protease. *Science*. 2003;300:1145–1148.

4   Lin W, Kim SS, Yeung E, et al. Hepatitis C virus core protein blocks interferon signaling by interaction with the STAT1 SH2 domain. *J Virol*. 2006;80:9226–9235.

5   Bode JG, Ludwig S, Ehrhardt C, et al. IFN-alpha antagonistic activity of HCV core protein involves induction of suppressor of cytokine signaling-3. *Faseb J.* 2003;17:488–490.

6   Polyak SJ, Khabar KS, Paschal DM, et al. Hepatitis C virus nonstructural 5A protein induces interleukin-8, leading to partial inhibition of the interferon-induced antiviral response. *J Virol.* 2001;75:6095–6106.

7   Gale MJ Jr, Korth MJ, Tang NM, et al. Evidence that hepatitis C virus resistance to interferon is mediated through repression of the PKR protein kinase by the nonstructural 5A protein. *Virology.* 1997;230:217–227.

8   Taylor DR, Shi ST, Romano PR, Barber GN, Lai MM. Inhibition of the interferon-inducible protein kinase PKR by HCV E2 protein. *Science.* 1999;285:107–110.

9   Topham NJ, Hewitt EW. Natural killer cell cytotoxicity: how do they pull the trigger? *Immunology.* 2009;128:7–15.

10 Jinushi M, Takehara T, Tatsumi T, et al. Negative regulation of NK cell activities by inhibitory receptor CD94/NKG2A leads to altered NK cell-induced modulation of dendritic cell functions in chronic hepatitis C virus infection. *J Immunol.* 2004;173:6072–6081.

11 Tseng CT, Klimpel GR. Binding of the hepatitis C virus envelope protein E2 to CD81 inhibits natural killer cell functions. *J Exp Med.* 2002;195:43–49.

12 Dolganiuc A, Chang S, Kodys K, et al. Hepatitis C virus (HCV) core protein-induced, monocyte-mediated mechanisms of reduced IFN-alpha and plasmacytoid dendritic cell loss in chronic HCV infection. *J Immunol.* 2006;177:6758–6768.

13 Dolganiuc A, Kodys K, Kopasz A, et al. Hepatitis C virus core and nonstructural protein 3 proteins induce pro- and anti-inflammatory cytokines and inhibit dendritic cell differentiation. *J Immunol.* 2003;170:5615–5624.

14 Auffermann-Gretzinger S, Keeffe EB, Levy S. Impaired dendritic cell maturation in patients with chronic, but not resolved, hepatitis C virus infection. *Blood.* 2001;97:3171–3176.

15 Thimme R, Bukh J, Spangenberg HC, et al. Viral and immunological determinants of hepatitis C virus clearance, persistence, and disease. *Proc Natl Acad Sci U S A.* 2002;99:15661–15668.

16 Logvinoff C, Major ME, Oldach D, et al. Neutralizing antibody response during acute and chronic hepatitis C virus infection. *Proc Natl Acad Sci U S A.* 2004;101:10149–10154.

17 Pestka JM, Zeisel MB, Bläser E, et al. Rapid induction of virus-neutralizing antibodies and viral clearance in a single-source outbreak of hepatitis C. *Proc Natl Acad Sci U S A.* 2007;104:6025–6030.

18 Semmo N, Lucas M, Krashias G, Lauer G, Chapel H, Klenerman P. Maintenance of HCV-specific T-cell responses in antibody-deficient patients a decade after early therapy. *Blood.* 2006;107:4570–4571.

19 Racanelli V, Frassanito MA, Leone P, et al. Antibody production and in vitro behavior of CD27-defined B-cell subsets: persistent hepatitis C virus infection changes the rules. *J Virol.* 2006;80:3923–3934.

20 Dammacco F, Sansonno D, Piccoli C, Racanelli V, D'Amore FP, Lauletta G. The lymphoid system in hepatitis C virus infection: autoimmunity, mixed cryoglobulinemia, and Overt B-cell malignancy. *Semin Liver Dis.* 2000;20:143–157.

21 Shoukry NH, Grakoui A, Houghton M, et al. Memory CD8+ T cells are required for protection from persistent hepatitis C virus infection. *J Exp Med.* 2003;197:1645–1655.

22 Grakoui A, Shoukry NH, Woollard DJ, et al. HCV persistence and immune evasion in the absence of memory T cell help. *Science.* 2003;302:659–662.

23 Diepolder HM, Zachoval R, Hoffmann RM, et al. Possible mechanism involving T-lymphocyte response to non-structural protein 3 in viral clearance in acute hepatitis C virus infection. *Lancet.* 1995;346:1006–1007.

24 von Hahn T, Yoon JC, Alter H, et al. Hepatitis C virus continuously escapes from neutralizing antibody and T-cell responses during chronic infection in vivo. *Gastroenterology.* 2007;132:667–678.

25 Helle F, Goffard A, Morel V, et al. The neutralizing activity of anti-hepatitis C virus antibodies is modulated by specific glycans on the E2 envelope protein. *J Virol.* 2007;81:8101–8111.

26 Radziewicz H, Ibegbu CC, Hon H, et al. Impaired hepatitis C virus (HCV)-specific effector CD8+ T cells undergo massive apoptosis in the peripheral blood during acute HCV infection and in the liver during the chronic phase of infection. *J Virol*. 2008;82:9808–9822.

27 Nakamoto N, Kaplan DE, Coleclough J, et al. Functional restoration of HCV-specific CD8 T cells by PD-1 blockade is defined by PD-1 expression and compartmentalization. *Gastroenterology*. 2008;134:1927–1937.

28 Bengsch B, Spangenberg HC, Kersting N, et al. Analysis of CD127 and KLRG1 expression on hepatitis C virus-specific CD8+ T cells reveals the existence of different memory T-cell subsets in the peripheral blood and liver. *J Virol*. 2007;81:945–953.

29 Boettler T, Spangenberg HC, Neumann-Haefelin C, et al. T cells with a CD4+CD25+ regulatory phenotype suppress in vitro proliferation of virus-specific CD8+ T cells during chronic hepatitis C virus infection. *J Virol*. 2005;79:7860–7867.

30 Cabrera R, Tu Z, Xu Y, et al. An immunomodulatory role for CD4(+)CD25(+) regulatory T lymphocytes in hepatitis C virus infection. *Hepatology*. 2004;40:1062–1071.

31 D'Ambrosio R, Aghemo A, Rumi MG, et al. A morphometric and immunohistochemical study to assess the benefit of a sustained virological response in hepatitis C virus patients with cirrhosis. *Hepatology*. 2012;56:532–543.

32 Heydtmann M, Adams DH. Chemokines in the immunopathogenesis of hepatitis C infection. *Hepatology*. 2009;49:676–688.

33 Clément S, Pascarella S, Conzelmann S, Gonelle-Gispert C, Guilloux K, Negro F. The hepatitis C virus core protein indirectly induces alpha-smooth muscle actin expression in hepatic stellate cells via interleukin-8. *J Hepatol*. 2010:52:635–643.

34 Ming-Ju H, Yih-Shou H, Tzy-Yen C, Hui-Ling C. Hepatitis C virus E2 protein induce reactive oxygen species (ROS)-related fibrogenesis in the HSC-T6 hepatic stellate cell line. *J Cell Biochem*. 2011;112:233–243.

35 Rüeger S, Bochud PY, Dufour JF, et al. Impact of common risk factors of fibrosis progression in chronic hepatitis C. *Gut*. 2014;64:1605–1615.

36 Asselah T, Rubbia-Brandt L, Marcellin P, Negro F. Steatosis in chronic hepatitis C: why does it really matter? *Gut*. 2006;55:123–130.

37 Rubbia-Brandt L, Quadri R, Abid K, et al. Hepatocyte steatosis is a cytopathic effect of hepatitis C virus genotype 3. *J Hepatol*. 2000;33:106–115.

38 Leandro G, Mangia A, Hui J, et al. Relationship between steatosis, inflammation, and fibrosis in chronic hepatitis C: a meta-analysis of individual patient data. *Gastroenterology*. 2006;130:1636–1642.

39 Waris G, Felmlee DJ, Negro F, Siddiqui A. Hepatitis C virus induces proteolytic cleavage of sterol regulatory element binding proteins and stimulates their phosphorylation via oxidative stress. *J Virol*. 2007;81:8122–8130.

40 Perlemuter G, Sabile A, Letteron P, et al. Hepatitis C virus core protein inhibits microsomal triglyceride transfer protein activity and very low density lipoprotein secretion: a model of viral-related steatosis. *Faseb J*. 2002;16:185–194.

41 Mirandola S, Realdon S, Iqbal J, et al. Liver microsomal triglyceride transfer protein is involved in hepatitis C liver steatosis. *Gastroenterology*. 2006;130:1661–1669.

42 de Gottardi A, Pazienza V, Pugnale P, et al. Peroxisome proliferator-activated receptor-alpha and -gamma mRNA levels are reduced in chronic hepatitis C with steatosis and genotype 3 infection. *Aliment Pharmacol Ther*. 2006;23:107–114.

43 Yamaguchi A, Tazuma S, Nishioka T, et al. Hepatitis C virus core protein modulates fatty acid metabolism and thereby causes lipid accumulation in the liver. *Dig Dis Sci*. 2005;50:1361–1371.

44 Dharancy S, Malapel M, Perlemuter G, et al. Impaired expression of the peroxisome proliferator-activated receptor alpha during hepatitis C virus infection. *Gastroenterology*. 2005;128:334–342.

45 Clément S, Peyrou M, Sanchez-Pareja A, et al. Down-regulation of phosphatase and tensin homolog by hepatitis C virus core 3a in hepatocytes triggers the formation of large lipid droplets. *Hepatology*. 2011;54:38–49.

46 Herker E, Ott M. Unique ties between hepatitis C virus replication and intracellular lipids. *Trends Endocrinol Metab*. 2011;22:241–248.

47 GBD 2013 Mortality and Causes of Death Collaborators. Global, regional, and national age-sex specific all-cause and cause-specific mortality for 240 causes of death, 1990–2013: a systematic analysis for the Global Burden of Disease Study 2013. *Lancet*. 2015;385:117–171.

48 Perz JF, Armstrong GL, Farrington LA, Hutin YJ, Bell BP. The contributions of hepatitis B virus and hepatitis C virus infections to cirrhosis and primary liver cancer worldwide. *J Hepatol*. 2006;45:529–538.

49 Simonetti RG, Cammà C, Fiorello F, Politi F, D'Amico G, Pagliaro L. Hepatocellular carcinoma. A worldwide problem and the major risk factors. *Dig Dis Sci*. 1991;36:962–972.

50 Hung CH, Wang JH, Hu TH, et al. Insulin resistance is associated with hepatocellular carcinoma in chronic hepatitis C infection. *World J Gastroenterol*. 2010;16:2265–2271.

51 Kuske L, Mensen A, Müllhaupt B, et al. Characteristics of patients with chronic hepatitis C who develop hepatocellular carcinoma. *Swiss Med Wkly*. 2012;142:w13651.

52 Ohata K, Hamasaki K, Toriyama K, et al. Hepatic steatosis is a risk factor for hepatocellular carcinoma in patients with chronic hepatitis C virus infection. *Cancer*. 2003;97:3036–3043.

53 Kurosaki M, Hosokawa T, Matsunaga K, et al. Hepatic steatosis in chronic hepatitis C is a significant risk factor for developing hepatocellular carcinoma independent of age, sex, obesity, fibrosis stage and response to interferon therapy. *Hepatol Res*. 2010;40:870–877.

54 Hayashi J, Aoki H, Kajino K, Moriyama M, Arakawa Y, Hino O. Hepatitis C virus core protein activates the MAPK/ERK cascade synergistically with tumor promoter TPA, but not with epidermal growth factor or transforming growth factor alpha. *Hepatology*. 2000;32:958–961.

55 Liu J, Ding X, Tang J, et al. Enhancement of canonical Wnt/beta-catenin signaling activity by HCV core protein promotes cell growth of hepatocellular carcinoma cells. *PLoS One*. 2011;6:e27496.

56 Taniguchi H, Kato N, Otsuka M, et al. Hepatitis C virus core protein upregulates transforming growth factor-beta 1 transcription. *J Med Virol*. 2004;72:52–59.

57 Higgs MR, Lerat H, Pawlotsky JM. Hepatitis C virus-induced activation of β-catenin promotes c-Myc expression and a cascade of pro-carcinogenetic events. *Oncogene*. 2013;32:4683–4693.

58 Hussain SP, Schwank J, Staib F, Wang XW, Harris CC. TP53 mutations and hepatocellular carcinoma: insights into the etiology and pathogenesis of liver cancer. *Oncogene*. 2007;26:2166–2176.

59 Nishimura T, Kohara M, Izumi K, et al. Hepatitis C virus impairs p53 via persistent overexpression of 3beta-hydroxysterol Delta24-reductase. *J Biol Chem*. 2009;284:36442–36452.

60 Munakata T, Nakamura M, Liang Y, Li K, Lemon SM. Down-regulation of the retinoblastoma tumor suppressor by the hepatitis C virus NS5B RNA-dependent RNA polymerase. *Proc Natl Acad Sci U S A*. 2005;102:18159–18164.

Chapter 5

Diagnosis

With the advent of highly active direct acting antivirals (DAAs) for the treatment of chronic hepatitis C, the goal of potential worldwide eradication of hepatitis C virus (HCV) infection seems achievable. However, it is becoming clear that one of the major challenges in reaching such a goal is the high rate of underdiagnosis of the infection and the insufficient link to care. In a US-based cohort carried out between 2001 and 2008, 30,140 patients from the National Health and Nutrition Examination Survey were tested for HCV infection; of those positive for HCV only half were aware of their HCV-positive status [1]. Similarly, in a French cross-sectional study by Meffre et al [2] 43% of HCV-positive individuals were unaware of their status. Underdiagnosis is partly due to the largely asymptomatic initial phase of chronic HCV infection, which can prevent early diagnosis and thus limit the potential benefits of antiviral drugs. In this context, the Centers for Disease Control and Prevention (CDC) recently recommend a population-based screening strategy based on birth cohorts. This method of screening is being considered by countries based on the success of the US birth cohort [3,4]. In this chapter we review the main aspects of the diagnosis of chronic HCV infection in accordance, where relevant, with major US and European guidelines.

Screening for chronic HCV infection

In light of evidence suggesting that risk factors in individuals diagnosed with HCV are under-reported, the CDC, the American Association for the Study of Liver Disease (AASLD), and the US Preventive Services Task Force

© Springer International Publishing Switzerland 2016   49
N. Goossens et al. (eds.), *Handbook of Hepatitis C*,
DOI 10.1007/978-3-319-28053-0_5

have implemented a one-time screening for HCV infection in all persons born between 1945 and 1965, the so-called 'baby-boomers' [3,5,6]. This strategy was supported by epidemiological findings in this age-group showing that baby-boomers accounted for approximately 75% of all HCV infections and had a five-fold higher prevalence of HCV than other age groups [3,5]. Early reports based on insurance claims in the US are encouraging as they indicate increased uptake of screening in this population (although the recommendation has yet to reach full penetration) [7]. Conversely, European guidelines recommend screening in targeted (higher risk) populations only and do not endorse population-wide screening [8].

US guidelines also endorse targeted HCV screening in at-risk individuals [5]. As the transmission of HCV is primarily through percutaneous exposure to contaminated blood, the CDC and AASLD-Infectious Disease Society of America (IDSA) guidelines [5] focus on risk exposure through injection drug use, health care exposure, incarceration, and potential vertical transmission though an HCV-positive mother (see Table 5.1 for a full list of risk factors that justify HCV screening). These recommendations pertain to the US setting and must be adapted to local risk factors, populations, and geographic considerations. Guidelines

1.	Individuals born between 1945 and 1965 irrespective of risk factors
2.	Risk behaviors
	A. Past or current injection drug use
	B. Intranasal drug use
3.	Risk exposures
	A. Long-term hemodialysis
	B. Tattoo in an unregulated setting
	C. Needle-stick, sharps, or mucosal exposure to HCV-infected blood in a healthcare setting
	D. Child born to HCV-infected mother

	E. Prior recipients of transfusions or organ transplants, including persons who:
	  – were notified that they received blood from a donor who later tested positive for HCV
	  – received a transfusion of blood or blood components, or underwent an organ transplant before July 1992
	  – received clotting factor concentrates produced before 1987

	F. Persons who were in prison
	G. HIV-infected individuals
	H. Unexplained liver disease or elevated aminotransferase levels
	I. Solid organ donors

Table 5.1 Recommendations for hepatitis C virus screening based on AASLD-IDSA, US Preventive Services Task Force, and CDC guidelines [5,6,9].

from the European Association for the Study of the Liver (EASL) are less specific and simply refer to "the local epidemiology of HCV infection, ideally within the framework of national plans" [8].

Assays for detecting HCV infection

The AASLD-IDSA and EASL guidelines suggest that individuals who qualify for HCV testing should sequentially be tested for HCV antibodies and, if positive, this should be followed by a confirmatory HCV RNA test [5,8] (Figure 5.1). In addition, genotype testing is mandatory if the patient will potentially qualify for therapy. Although modern diagnostic assays for HCV are highly accurate, their limitations must be known and understood by the clinician in order to minimize medical costs and to avoid unnecessary psychological burden on screened persons.

Serology

Currently, the most widely used assay for initial screening is a third-generation enzyme immunoassay (EIA) that detects structural and non-structural (NS) viral proteins. Third-generation EIAs detect antibodies

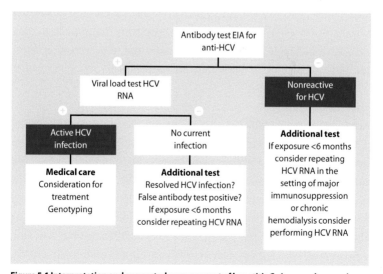

Figure 5.1 Interpretation and suggested management of hepatitis C virus serology and RNA results. In general these guidelines are consistent with those published by the US Center for Disease Control and Prevention [10]. EIA, enzyme immunoassay; HCV, hepatitis C virus; RNA, ribonucleic acid.

that bind to recombinant antigens derived from four viral regions: core, NS3, NS4, and NS5. Current serologic assays are highly specific (>99%), but the positive predictive value may actually be low in populations with low HCV prevalence, such as screening of volunteer blood donors or of the general population, resulting in a considerable number of false-positive results in these settings [11]. Sensitivity of HCV EIAs is high, approximately 98% [12]; however false-negatives may occur in the setting of major immunosuppression, chronic hemodialysis, or acute HCV infection prior to seroconversion.

Rapid antibody testing

Due to an increasing demand for rapid point-of-care diagnostic tests for HCV, the US Food and Drug Administration (FDA) approved the OraQuick® HCV Rapid Antibody Test in 2011 for use with whole blood samples obtained either by venipuncture or finger-stick capillary blood. The results from this point-of-care test are available in 20–40 minutes; however, a positive test should be followed up with supplementary HCV testing. Diagnostic performance of this test is similar to that of EIAs, with pooled sensitivity and specificity of >99% according to a recent systematic review by Khuroo et al [12], suggesting that, thanks to their ease of use and rapid results, these tests could lead to wider testing access for those at risk of HCV (dependent on cost).

HCV RNA testing

According to the AASLD-IDSA guidelines [5], the indications for testing with an HCV nucleic acid test include a positive HCV serology (to confirm current active HCV infection), patients who are immunocompromised (including those on chronic hemodialysis) even if HCV serology is negative, or individuals exposed to HCV within the last 6 months who may not have developed detectable HCV antibodies. In addition, HCV RNA testing should be performed in all patients with HCV undergoing treatment with antiviral therapy and at regular intervals during and after treatment [5].

Qualitative and quantitative HCV RNA assays

Qualitative assays do not allow quantification of viral HCV RNA titers but they provide a categorical yes or no answer to whether HCV RNA is detectable in the sample. Historically, qualitative assays were used for HCV diagnosis due to increased sensitivity. However, current ultrasensitive quantitative HCV RNA assays achieve similar sensitivity to qualitative assays, and have a lower limit of detection (around 10 IU/mL).

Genotyping HCV

HCV has a high degree of genetic heterogeneity that has significantly complicated classification. Genotypes (equidistant phylogenetic groups) differ from each other by 31–33% of nucleotides, and the next level of classification, subtypes, differ by 20–25% of nucleotides [13]. Nevertheless, despite this sequence diversity, all HCV genotypes share an identical complement of co-linear genes of similar size in the large open reading frame. The most recent classification scheme has identified seven distinct genotypes, 67 confirmed subtypes, and 20 provisionally assigned subtypes [14]. Clinically, genotyping HCV is critical as it determines the type and response to antiviral therapy. Additionally, HCV genotype, in particular genotype 3, has also been linked to differing prognosis and histological findings [15]. EASL guidelines recommend an assay specifically distinguishing genotype 1a and 1b, as the result affects the antiviral regimen chosen [8].

Technically, HCV genotyping is performed by a number of different methods. The gold standard is the direct sequencing of the viral genome with phylogenetic analysis. Alternative methods more suitable for routine clinical use involve sequencing only the 5`UTR of the viral genome or differential hybridization of the same region to oligonucleotides immobilized on nitrocellulose strips [16]. Differentiation between subtypes 1a and 1b, especially in the setting of treatment with DAAs, is relevant and methods solely based on the analysis of the 5`UTR failed to identify subtype 1a in approximately 25% of samples, prompting the development of a reverse hybridization assay targeting the 5`UTR and core-coding region [17]. This method allows correct classification of subtypes 1a and 1b in more than 99% of cases [17].

Liver biopsy and histology

One of the most important steps in the management of the individual patient with chronic HCV is the assessment of the stage of liver disease and in particular the assessment for the presence of advanced fibrosis, as underlined in the AASLD-IDSA and EASL guidelines [5,8]. The reference standard for the assessment of hepatic disease activity and staging has traditionally been liver biopsy, although, recently a number of non-invasive alternatives have been made available in selected individuals.

Liver biopsy, most often performed through the right intercostal percutaneous route, allows the assessment of the grade of hepatic injury (necroinflammatory activity) and the stage of disease (fibrosis stage or cirrhosis) (Figure 5.2).

Numerous grading and staging systems have been developed in an effort to quantify and uniformize the assessment of liver disease severity; two of the most common systems are the Ishak [18] and the METAVIR systems [19]. The necroinflammatory component schematically combines, depending on the score, piecemeal necrosis (periportal or periseptal interface hepatitis), lobular activity, confluent necrosis, and

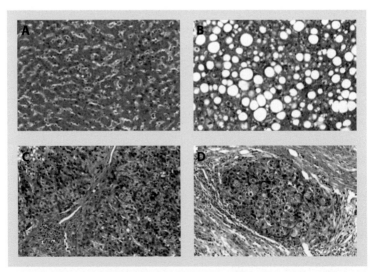

Figure 5.2 Illustrative histological photomicrographs of healthy liver, steatosis, fibrosis, and cirrhosis. A, healthy liver; B, steatosis; C, fibrosis; d, cirrhosis. The top two panels are hematoxylin and eosin stained and the bottom two are trichrome stained.

portal inflammation and yields a histological grading score of 0–18 in the Ishak system and a simpler 0–3 activity score in the METAVIR system. The fibrosis staging score assesses the degree of portal fibrosis and the presence of fibrotic septa formation and is staged 0–6 and 0–4 in the Ishak and METAVIR systems, respectively (Table 5.2). In addition, liver biopsy may identify other hepatic lesions, such as signs of alcoholic and non-alcoholic fatty liver disease, iron deposits, or other findings suggesting potential cofactors to HCV disease progression that are useful in the management of the patient. Finally, another advantage of histology is the possibility to perform additional, more advanced analyses, such as specific histological staining or molecular analyses that inform on the risk of disease progression above commonly identified clinical risk factors [20]. However, one must also take into account the potential limitations of staging liver disease using hepatic histology, underlined in studies comparing fibrosis assessment of entire surgical samples and virtual biopsies in the same samples and showing that biopsy samples less than 25 mm were associated with an increased variability of fibrosis assessment [21]. In addition, potential side effects and risks associated with liver biopsy must also be taken into account. In a French prospective nationwide survey of over 2000 liver biopsies, although no deaths related to the procedure were noted, severe complications were observed in 0.57% of patients and were associated with number

Stage	Ishak system	METAVIR system
0	No fibrosis	No fibrosis
1	Fibrous expansion of some portal areas	Stellate enlargement of portal tract but without septa formation
2	Fibrous expansion of most portal areas	Enlargement of portal tract with rare septa formation
3	Fibrous expansion of most portal areas with occasional portal to portal bridging	Numerous septa formation
4	Fibrous expansion of portal areas with marked bridging as well as portal to central	Cirrhosis
5	Marked bridging fibrosis with occasional nodules (incomplete cirrhosis)	N/A
6	Probably/definite cirrhosis	N/A

Table 5.2 Comparison of fibrosis staging in the Ishak scoring system and the METAVIR system [18,19]. N/A indicates not applicable.

of passes (number of biopsies taken), inexperience of the operator, not using US guidance, and not using atropine [22]. However, this study may have been underpowered to identify death after liver biopsy, as a large multicenter retrospective review [23] of over 65,000 percutaneous liver biopsies in Italy reported that, although infrequent, death occurred in 9 per 100,000 cases. The study also demonstrated that Menghini's needle, currently recommended for routine biopsy, was associated with fewer complications [23]. Pain is a common but less threatening side effect of liver biopsy and is present in approximately one-third of patients. Other routes of access to hepatic tissue in patients at risk of hemorrhage or complications include transjugular liver biopsy [24], which may reduce the risk of complications; however, this is costly, requires experienced personnel, and is only available in a limited number of centers.

Non-invasive tests

Due to potential complications and risks of sampling bias of liver biopsy, a significant effort has been devoted to developing non-invasive strategies to assess liver disease severity in the context of HCV infection. A number of different scores, using a combination of various clinical parameters and serum markers, have been developed especially to assess the degree of liver fibrosis [25]. Schematically, serum-based biomarkers may be differentiated into direct markers (reflecting deposition and removal of extracellular matrix within the liver, such as serum hyaluronate, laminin, type IV collagen, and procollagen) and indirect markers (such as prothrombin time, platelet count, and ratio of aspartate aminotransferase [AST] to alanine aminotransferase [ALT]). Markers are often combined in tests that have been validated, such as the AST to platelet ratio index (APRI) [26], fibrosis-4 (FIB-4) [27], Forns index [28], Lok index [29] (based on the HALT-C cohort), or the FibroTest (FibroSURE™ in the US) [30]. Performance of these assays varies widely, with reported sensitivities of 30–98% and specificities of 45–99% [25]. Non-invasive tests often perform well for detecting advanced fibrosis and cirrhosis; however, their diagnostic performance is less clear for intermediate levels of fibrosis. In addition, their usefulness at determining response to therapy and patient prognosis is still under investigation.

Transient elastography (TE) (also known as FibroScan®) is a 'physical' approach to non-invasively assess liver fibrosis by measuring liver stiffness. Advantages of TE include:

- short procedure time;
- immediate results; and
- relative ease for learning or performing the procedure.

However, although very good inter- and intra-observer agreement has been noted, a measurement cannot be obtained in approximately 20% of individuals with the regular probe [31]. A newer (extra-large) probe seems to resolve some of these issues, at least in obese individuals [32]. Nevertheless, similar to serum-based markers, TE accurately distinguishes patients with advanced fibrosis from those with no or very early fibrosis; however, its performance is insufficient in patients with intermediate grades of fibrosis [25]. Newer strategies, such as Acoustic Radiation Force Impulse Imaging (ARFI), are currently being evaluated and compared to more established non-invasive strategies [33].

A combination of non-invasive strategies has been shown to increase overall performance and possibly reduce the need for liver biopsy in selected patients. For instance, a large study by Boursier et al [34] of more than 1700 patients with hepatitis C found that a combination of FibroMeter® and FibroScan® accurately stratified patients into six fibrosis classes and eliminated the requirement for liver biopsy, although these findings require further validation.

Conclusion

In conclusion, many tools are available to clinicians to accurately diagnose, risk stratify, and stage a patient with suspected HCV infection. Efforts are now underway to improve screening and identification of HCV-infected patients, and the current tools available for diagnosis and risk assessment will probably require refinement to further streamline the management of patients.

Key points

- Underdiagnosis of HCV infection and insufficient link to care are major challenges that need to be addressed in order to achieve the goal of global HCV eradication.

- The initial phase of chronic HCV infection is largely asymptomatic, which prevents early diagnosis and limits the potential benefits of antiviral drugs.

- At-risk individuals should be sequentially tested for HCV antibodies and, if positive, followed-up with a confirmatory HCV RNA test.

- Genotyping HCV is critical as it determines response to antiviral therapy. The gold standard is the direct sequencing of the viral genome with phylogenetic analysis.

- HCV nucleic acid testing should be carried out in individuals with positive HCV serology, those who are immunocompromised, individuals recently exposed to HCV, and in all patients with HCV undergoing treatment.

- Assessment of the stage of liver disease and the presence of advanced fibrosis is one of the most important steps in management of patients with chronic HCV.

- The grade of hepatic injury and the stage of disease have traditionally been assessed by liver biopsy.

- Recently, a number of non-invasive alternatives have been made available in selected individuals:

    - direct and indirect serum-based biomarkers combined in validated tests (eg, APRI, FIB-4, Forns index, Lok index, and FibroTest); and

    - physical approaches (eg, measuring liver stiffness using TE).

References

1   Denniston MM, Klevens RM, McQuillan GM, Jiles RB. Awareness of infection, knowledge of hepatitis C, and medical follow-up among individuals testing positive for hepatitis C: National Health and Nutrition Examination Survey 2001–2008. *Hepatology*. 2012;55:1652–1661.

2   Meffre C, Le Strat Y, Delarocque-Astagneau E, et al. Prevalence of hepatitis B and hepatitis C virus infections in France in 2004: social factors are important predictors after adjusting for known risk factors. *J Med Virol*. 2010;82:546–555.

3   Smith BD, Morgan RL, Beckett GA, et al. Recommendations for the identification of chronic hepatitis C virus infection among persons born during 1945–1965. *MMWR Recomm Rep*. 2012;61:1–32.

4   Grebely J, Bilodeau M, Feld, JJ, et al. The second Canadian symposium on hepatitis C virus: a call to action. *Can J Gastroenterol*. 2013;27:627–632.

5   AASLD/IDSA HCV Guidance Panel. Hepatitis C guidance: AASLD-IDSA recommendations for testing, managing, and treating adults infected with hepatitis C virus. *Hepatology*. 2015;62:932–954.

6   Moyer VA, US Preventive Services Task Force. Screening for hepatitis C virus infection in adults: US Preventive Services Task Force recommendation statement. *Ann Intern Med*. 2013;159:349–357.

7   Coyle J, Brousseau G, George E, Eckel S, Macomber K. Evaluation of CDC's Hepatitis C Birth-Cohort Screening Recommendation Using Medical Claims Data. The Council of State and Territorial Epidemiologists (CSTE) Annual Conference. June 14–18, 2015; Boston, US.

8   European Association for Study of Liver. EASL Recommendations on Treatment of Hepatitis C 2015. *J Hepatol*. 2015;63:199–236.

9   Centers for Disease Control and Prevention (CDC). Testing for HCV infection: an update of guidance for clinicians and laboratorians. *MMWR Morb Mortal Wkly Rep*. 2013;62:362–365.

10 Alter HJ, Aragon T, AuBuchon JP, et al. Recommendations for prevention and control of hepatitis C virus (HCV) infection and HCV-related chronic disease. Centers for Disease Control and Prevention. *MMWR Recomm Rep*. 1998;47:1–39.

11 Alter MJ, Kuhnert WL, Finelli L. Centers for Disease Control and Prevention. Guidelines for laboratory testing and result reporting of antibody to hepatitis C virus. Centers for Disease Control and Prevention. *MMWR Recomm Rep*. 2003;52:1–13.

12 Khuroo MS, Khuroo NS, Khuroo MS. Diagnostic accuracy of point-of-care tests for hepatitis C virus infection: a systematic review and meta-analysis. *PLoS One*. 2015;10:e0121450.

13 Simmonds P, Bukh J, Combet C, et al. Consensus proposals for a unified system of nomenclature of hepatitis C virus genotypes. *Hepatology*. 2005;42:962–973.

14 Smith DB, Bukh J, Kuiken C, et al. Expanded classification of hepatitis C virus into 7 genotypes and 67 subtypes: updated criteria and genotype assignment web resource. *Hepatology*. 2014;59:318–327.

15 Goossens N, Negro F. Is genotype 3 of the hepatitis C virus the new villain? *Hepatology*. 2014;59:2403–2412.

16 Stuyver L, Wyseur A, van Arnhem W, Hernandez F, Maertens G. Second-generation line probe assay for hepatitis C virus genotyping. *J Clin Microbiol*. 1996;34:2259–2266.

17 Chevaliez S, Bouvier-Alias M, Brillet R, Pawlotsky JM. Hepatitis C virus (HCV) genotype 1 subtype identification in new HCV drug development and future clinical practice. *PLoS One*. 2009;4:e8209.

18 Ishak K, Baptista A, Bianchi L, et al. Histological grading and staging of chronic hepatitis. *J Hepatol*. 1995;22:696–699.

19 Bedossa P, Poynard T. An algorithm for the grading of activity in chronic hepatitis C. The METAVIR Cooperative Study Group. *Hepatology*. 1996;24:289–293.

20 King LY, Canasto-Chibuque C, Johnson KB. A genomic and clinical prognostic index for hepatitis C-related early-stage cirrhosis that predicts clinical deterioration. *Gut*. 2015;64:1296–1302.

21   Bedossa P, Dargère D, Paradis V. Sampling variability of liver fibrosis in chronic hepatitis C. *Hepatology*. 2003;38:1449–1457.

22   Cadranel JF, Rufat P, Degos F. Practices of liver biopsy in France: results of a prospective nationwide survey. For the Group of Epidemiology of the French Association for the Study of the Liver (AFEF). *Hepatology*. 2000;32:477–481.

23   Piccinino F, Sagnelli E, Pasquale G, Giusti G. Complications following percutaneous liver biopsy. A multicentre retrospective study on 68,276 biopsies. *J Hepatol*. 1986;2:165–173.

24   Ble M, Procopet B, Miquel R, Hernandez-Gea V, García-Pagán. Transjugular liver biopsy. *Clin Liver Dis*. 2014;18:767–778.

25   Castera L. Noninvasive methods to assess liver disease in patients with hepatitis B or C. *Gastroenterology*. 2012;142:1293–1302.

26   Wai CT, Greenson JK, Fontana RJ, et al. A simple noninvasive index can predict both significant fibrosis and cirrhosis in patients with chronic hepatitis C. *Hepatology*. 2003;38:518–526.

27   Vallet-Pichard A, Mallet V, Nalpas B, et al. FIB-4: an inexpensive and accurate marker of fibrosis in HCV infection. Comparison with liver biopsy and fibrotest. *Hepatology*. 2007;46:32–36.

28   Forns X, Ampurdanès S, Llovet JM, et al. Identification of chronic hepatitis C patients without hepatic fibrosis by a simple predictive model. Hepatology. 2002;36:986–992.

29   Lok AS, Ghany MG, Goodman ZD, et al. Predicting cirrhosis in patients with hepatitis C based on standard laboratory tests: results of the HALT-C cohort. *Hepatology*. 2005;42:282–292.

30   Imbert-Bismut F, Ratziu V, Pieroni L, et al. Biochemical markers of liver fibrosis in patients with hepatitis C virus infection: a prospective study. *Lancet*. 2001;357:1069–1075.

31   Castéra L, Foucher J, Bernard PH, et al. Pitfalls of liver stiffness measurement: A 5-year prospective study of 13,369 examinations. *Hepatology*. 2010;51:828–835.

32   Myers RP, Pomier-Layrargues G, Kirsch R, et al. Feasibility and diagnostic performance of the FibroScan XL probe for liver stiffness measurement in overweight and obese patients. *Hepatology*. 2012;55:199–208.

33   Rizzo L, Calvaruso V, Cacopardo B, et al. Comparison of transient elastography and acoustic radiation force impulse for non-invasive staging of liver fibrosis in patients with chronic hepatitis C. *Am J Gastroenterol*. 2011;106:2112–2120.

34   Boursier J, de Ledinghen V, Zarski JP. Comparison of eight diagnostic algorithms for liver fibrosis in hepatitis C: new algorithms are more precise and entirely noninvasive. *Hepatology*. 2012;55:58–67.

Chapter 6

Management of HCV infection

Introduction

There has been a tremendous shift in the landscape of hepatitis C virus (HCV) management with the advent of direct acting antivirals (DAAs). HCV therapy with DAAs has dramatically increased the efficacy of therapy, reduced side effects, and reduced treatment duration. However, due to high pricing strategies, this progress has come at a high financial cost, limiting the accessibility of these novel drugs to patients with advanced stages of hepatitis C. This state of affairs raises important societal and ethical issues [1]. In this chapter, we review the current management strategies of patients with HCV infection in light of major international guidelines.

Goals of therapy

The primary goal of the management of patients with HCV is to reduce or eliminate the complications of chronic HCV infection, such as the development of cirrhosis, hepatic decompensation, hepatocellular carcinoma (HCC), extrahepatic manifestations, and death. To achieve this goal, the endpoint of therapy, or the cure of HCV, is defined as sustained virological response (SVR) (undetectable HCV RNA at 12 weeks [SVR12] or 24 weeks [SVR24] after treatment completion). SVR has been associated with reduced all-cause mortality, reduced liver-related mortality and transplantation, and reduced development of HCC [2]; reinforcing its role as a robust endpoint of antiviral therapy.

© Springer International Publishing Switzerland 2016
N. Goossens et al. (eds.), *Handbook of Hepatitis C*,
DOI 10.1007/978-3-319-28053-0_6

Patient assessment for antiviral therapy

As a general rule, all patients with evidence of virological presence of HCV (ie, detectable blood HCV levels) should be assessed for possible antiviral therapy. Every patient considered for antiviral therapy should have a complete history recorded in their medical records. The history should focus on the presence or absence of symptoms related to liver disease or extrahepatic manifestations and, additionally, previous antiviral treatment history should be clarified (the pattern of response to previous therapy allows categorization of patients based on their treatment history) (Box 6.1).

Assessment of liver fibrosis is a key component of patient evaluation as the prognosis of patients and their response to antiviral therapy is strongly correlated with the stage of fibrosis (see Chapter 3). As discussed previously, although liver biopsy has traditionally been considered the gold standard to define the fibrosis stage, current guidelines endorse non-invasive strategies (including liver stiffness measurement and blood biomarkers) and suggest liver biopsy only in cases where there is uncertainty or potential additional etiologies of liver disease [3].

HCV viral RNA load and especially HCV genotyping and subtyping of genotype 1a from 1b are key factors that will indicate treatment strategy. HCV resistance testing at the outset is not recommended, unless considering a regimen of pegylated interferon-alpha (peg-IFN-α), ribavirin, and simeprevir in patients with HCV genotype 1 (due to reduced responsiveness of Q80K mutated strains in genotype 1a HCV infection) [3,4].

Indications and contraindications to antiviral therapy

Major international guidelines recommend that all patients with chronic HCV infection be considered for antiviral therapy [3,4]. However, due to limited financial and human resources, treatment should be prioritized

---

Box 6.1 Key definitions in the categorization of patient treatment history

- Treatment-naïve patients are those who have never received antiviral therapy.
- Relapse patients are those with undetectable HCV RNA at the end of treatment but relapse after the end of therapy without achieving an SVR.
- Non-responders are patients who fail to achieve a decline of 2 $\log_{10}$ HCV RNA (IU/mL) after 12 weeks of therapy with an interferon-based regimen, or failure to achieve undetectable HCV RNA during 24 weeks of therapy.

based on fibrosis stage, degree of liver failure, risk of progression to advanced disease, presence of extrahepatic manifestations, and risk of HCV transmission. The highest priority is assigned to patients with HCV with METAVIR stage F3 fibrosis or compensated cirrhosis, liver transplant recipients, and patients with severe extrahepatic manifestations (such as essential mixed cryoglobulinemia with end-organ manifestations and renal manifestations of HCV infection) [5,6]. In addition, The European Association for the Study of the Liver (EASL) guidelines [3] endorse urgent treatment of patients with decompensated cirrhosis with interferon (IFN)-free regimens. A high priority to HCV therapy is also assigned to individuals with HCV and human immunodeficiency virus (HIV) or hepatitis B virus (HBV) co-infection (regardless of fibrosis stage), patients with debilitating fatigue, co-existent liver disease, or type 2 diabetes mellitus. Patients with METAVIR stage F2 fibrosis are also assigned a high priority to therapy in the American Association for the Study of Liver Diseases/Infectious Diseases Society of America (AASLD-IDSA) guidelines [4]; however, therapy should be individualized and may be postponed in patients with F0–F1 fibrosis and none of the above-mentioned complications. Another group that should be prioritized for therapy regardless of fibrosis stage is individuals at risk of transmitting HCV as treatment may lead to potential transmission reduction benefits [3,4]. This group includes men who have sex with men (who are HIV positive), individuals who have high-risk sexual practices, active injection drug users, patients on hemodialysis, HCV-infected women of childbearing age wishing to get pregnant, HCV-infected health care workers performing exposure-prone procedures, and incarcerated individuals.

In general, antiviral therapy is contraindicated in patients with limited life expectancy (due to non-HCV-related comorbidities) who would therefore not benefit from therapy, although, every individual case must be assessed by an experienced clinician. Specific contraindications to antiviral therapy essentially include contraindications to specific drugs, for example, therapy with peg-IFN-α and ribavirin is absolutely contraindicated in patients with severe uncontrolled depression, psychosis or epilepsy, pregnant women, decompensated liver disease, severe comorbid medical disease, or patients with severe neutropenia and/or thrombocytopenia. As of 2015, no known absolute contraindications to DAAs have been described, although, sofosbuvir is contraindicated in severe renal failure and the safety of several DAAs in certain clinical situations (such as decompensated liver disease) remains unknown. In addition, the clinician is encouraged to assess all potential drug interactions, especially in the setting of antiretroviral therapy for HIV.

Overview of drugs currently approved for HCV management

Interferon and ribavirin

The combination of peg-IFN-α and ribavirin was the cornerstone of HCV treatment until 2011, when more effective, novel DAAs were introduced (Figure 6.1). Treatment lasted 24–48 weeks depending on the viral genotype and severity of liver disease. This regimen led to SVR rates of approximately 40–50% in patients with genotype 1 and 4, and higher SVR rates in patients with genotype 2, 3, 5, and 6 [7,8]. Side effects of this regimen are substantial and include anemia, neutropenia, thrombocytopenia, fatigue, neuropsychiatric effects, flu-like symptoms, and

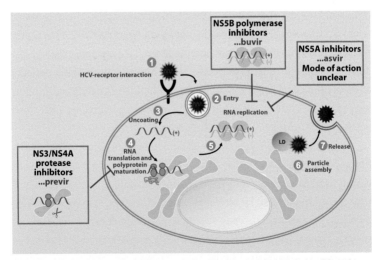

Figure 6.1 Therapeutic targets of direct acting antivirals in the hepatitis C virus life cycle.
The suffix of the name of the different drugs indicates its target: NS3/4A protease inhibitors end with the suffix 'previr', NS5A inhibitors end with 'asvir', and NS5B polymerase inhibitors end with 'buvir'. HCV, hepatitis C virus; LD, lipid; NS, non-structural; RNA, ribonucleic acid.

multiple other symptoms. Discontinuation/interruption of therapy due to side effects and contraindications occurs in 10–20% of patients [8].

NS3/4A protease inhibitors

Non-structural (NS)3/4A protease inhibitors (PIs) inhibit the viral NS3/4A serine protease by blocking the NS3 catalytic site or the NS3/NS4A interaction. In 2011, two first generation NS3/4A PIs, telaprevir and boceprevir, were licensed for use in genotype 1 HCV infection in conjunction with peg-IFN-α and ribavirin. SVR rates for this new combination improved to approximately 70% [9,10]; however, the side effect profile of first generation PIs (especially in patients with advanced fibrosis) as well as the pill burden has limited their use since the availability of better tolerated, more efficacious alternatives.

Simeprevir, a second generation NS3/4A PI, was approved in the EU and the US in 2014. It has been shown to be effective in patients with HCV genotype 1 in association with peg-IFN-α and ribavirin, although it should not be used for patients with prior failure of PI. Simeprevir is most efficacious in treatment-naïve patients and patients with prior relapses [11,12]; SVR rates are lower in patients with cirrhosis and treatment-experienced patients who had prior partial or null response [11–13]. Nevertheless, despite an improved side effect profile, the use of combination simeprevir- and peg-IFN-α-based therapy remains limited due to the side effects linked to IFN. A combination of simeprevir and the NS5B inhibitor, sofosbuvir, has been shown to be effective in patients with genotype 1, based on the COSMOS (NCT01466790) and OPTIMIST (NCT02114177, NCT02114151) trials [14,15]. Simeprevir is generally well tolerated, although photosensitivity and rash have been reported, and due to hepatic elimination of simeprevir it is contraindicated in the setting of liver failure (Child-Turcotte-Pugh class B or C). In addition, drug interactions should be checked prior to administering this drug as it is metabolized by the CYP3A family.

Paritaprevir is a PI used in combination with low-dose ritonavir for pharmacological boosting and is currently combined with ombitasvir, an NS5A inhibitor, and usually dasabuvir, a NS5B inhibitor (except in case of infection with genotype 4).

NS5A inhibitors

NS5A inhibitors inhibit the NS5A protein, which plays a key role in HCV replication and assembly. These molecules are generally potent and have a pan-genotypic activity, but a low barrier to resistance means that viral resistance can develop relatively easily. Currently, approved members of this class include ledipasvir, daclatasvir, and ombitasvir.

Daclatasvir and ledipasvir are generally used in combination with sofosbuvir, whereas ombitasvir is available as a fixed-dose combination with paritaprevir and ritonavir, usually also with dasabuvir. NS5A inhibitors have few reported side effects, although, there is a risk for drug interactions; daclatasvir, for example, is metabolized through CYP3A4 and should not be administered with inducers/inhibitors of this cytochrome without dosage adjustment.

NS5B inhibitors

The NS5B viral protein is a RNA-dependent RNA polymerase that is required for HCV replication. NS5B inhibitors are active across all genotypes due to the highly conserved nature of the RNA polymerase. NS5B inhibitors are separated into two classes; nucleoside PIs (including sofosbuvir) and non-nucleoside PIs (such as dasabuvir).

Sofosbuvir was the first NS5B inhibitor approved for HCV therapy (approved in the US and EU in 2014 for use in combination therapy). Its excretion is primarily renal so it should be avoided or reduced in patients with severe renal impairment. No dose adjustment is required in patients with hepatic impairment. Reported side effects are generally mild and include fatigue, nausea, and anemia, although, these symptoms may be attributable to concomitant peg-IFN-α and ribavirin use. Recently, cases of symptomatic bradycardia in patients on sofosbuvir therapy have been reported, although, it remains unclear what the clinical consequences of these findings are [16]. Although sofosbuvir is not metabolized by cytochrome P450, it is transported by permeability glycoprotein (P-gp) and therapeutic levels may be affected by P-gp inducers such as rifampin, carbamazepine, or phenytoin.

As a class, non-nucleoside NS5B inhibitors are less potent, have more genotype specificity, and a lower barrier to resistance. Dasabuvir is generally added to ombitasvir, paritaprevir, and ritonavir.

Treatment regimens for chronic HCV

The following sections summarize the antiviral treatment regimens for patients with HCV; however, the reader must be aware that there is a constant evolution in available antiviral therapies and that part of these recommendations may be outdated at the time of reading. Therefore, the reader is encouraged to consult the most current international [3,4] and national treatment guidelines and consult with local experts before selecting the appropriate therapy for the individual patient.

Treatment regimens discussed here are broadly in agreement with guidelines from EASL and AASLD-IDSA [3,4]. Treatment guidelines for treatment-naïve patients with chronic HCV infection are summarized in Table 6.1, where key commonalities and differences between EU and US guidelines are highlighted [5,6,11,14,17–27].

Genotype 1

A number of options are currently available for the treatment of HCV genotype 1 infection. Peg-IFN-α-containing regimens include combinations of peg-IFN-α, ribavirin, and sofosbuvir [19] or peg-IFN-α, ribavirin, and simeprevir [11]. The combination of peg-IFN-α, ribavirin, and sofosbuvir for 12 weeks in treatment-naïve patients was shown to achieve high SVR rates in non-cirrhotic and cirrhotic patients alike (SVR 92% and 80%, respectively) in the NEUTRINO trial (NCT01641640) [19]. Although prospective Phase III data of SVR rates in patients who previously failed peg-IFN-α ribavirin therapy is lacking, real-world experience in a diverse, longitudinal observational cohort including 45% treatment-experienced patients has shown SVR4 rates of 90% and 70% in non-cirrhotic and cirrhotic patients, respectively [28]. The PI-based combination of peg-IFN-α, ribavirin, and simeprevir was evaluated in the QUEST clinical trials (NCT01289782 and NCT01290679), with overall SVR rates of approximately 80% in treatment-naïve patients [11,12]. However, this combination requires total therapy duration of 24–48 weeks, is less effective than sofosbuvir-based regimens, not recommended in genotype 1a patients with the Q80K substitution polymorphism, and SVR rates of only 60% were achieved in patients with cirrhosis. Interestingly, although EASL guidelines maintain the recommendation for peg-IFN-α-based therapy

Patient group	HCV genotype	EASL guidelines	AASLD-IDSA guidelines	Reference
Non-cirrhotic patients	1	Ledipasvir + sofosbuvir for 12 weeks	Yes	[17]
		Paritaprevir/ritonavir/ombitasvir + dasabuvir (+ ribavirin if genotype 1a) for 12 weeks	Yes	[18]
		Sofosbuvir + peg-IFN-α + ribavirin for 12 weeks	No	[19]
		Simeprevir + peg-IFN-α + ribavirin for 12 weeks followed by peg-IFN-α + ribavirin for 12 additional weeks	No	[11]
		Simeprevir + sofosbuvir for 12 weeks	Yes	[14]
		Sofosbuvir + daclatasvir for 12 weeks	Yes	[20]
	2	Sofosbuvir + ribavirin for 12 weeks	Yes	[19]
	3	Sofosbuvir + peg-IFN-α + ribavirin for 12 weeks	Yes	[21]
		Sofosbuvir + ribavirin for 24 weeks	Yes, alternative	[22]
		Sofosbuvir + daclatasvir for 12 weeks	Yes	[23]
	4	Sofosbuvir + peg-IFN-α + ribavirin for 12 weeks	Yes, alternative	[19]
		Simeprevir + peg-IFN-α + ribavirin for 12 weeks followed by peg-IFN-α + ribavirin for 12 additional weeks	No	[24]
		Ledipasvir + sofosbuvir for 12 weeks	Yes	[25]
		Paritaprevir/ritonavir/ombitasvir + ribavirin for 12 weeks	Yes	[5]
		Simeprevir + sofosbuvir for 12 weeks	No	[14]
		Sofosbuvir + daclatasvir for 12 weeks	No	

Table 6.1 Hepatitis C virus treatment regimens recommended in treatment-naïve patients with genotypes 1–4, with comparison between EASL and AASLD-IDSA guidelines [5,6,11,14,17–27] (continued on next page).

Patient group	HCV genotype	EASL guidelines	AASLD-IDSA guidelines	Reference
Cirrhotic patients	1	Ledipasvir + sofosbuvir + ribavirin for 12 weeks	Ledipasvir + sofosbuvir for 12 weeks	[17]
		Paritaprevir/ritonavir/ ombitasvir + dasabuvir + ribavirin for 12 (genotype 1b) or 24 (genotype 1a) weeks	Yes	[6]
		Sofosbuvir + peg-IFN-α + ribavirin for 12 weeks	No	[19]
		Simeprevir + peg-IFN-α + ribavirin for 12 weeks followed by peg-IFN-α + ribavirin for 12 additional weeks	No	[11]
		Simeprevir + sofosbuvir + ribavirin for 12 weeks	Genotype 1a: simeprevir + sofosbuvir +/- ribavirin for 24 weeks (no Q80K polymorphism)	[14]
			Genotype 1b: simeprevir + sofosbuvir +/- ribavirin for 24 weeks	
		Sofosbuvir + daclatasvir + ribavirin for 12 weeks	Sofosbuvir + daclatasvir +/- ribavirin for 24 weeks	[20]
	2	Sofosbuvir + ribavirin for 16–20 weeks	Sofosbuvir + ribavirin for 16 weeks	[26]
		Sofosbuvir + peg-IFN-α + ribavirin for 12 weeks	No	[27]
		Sofosbuvir + daclatasvir for 12 weeks	Yes	[20]
	3	Sofosbuvir + peg-IFN-α + ribavirin for 12 weeks	Yes	[27]
		Sofosbuvir + ribavirin for 24 weeks	Yes, alternative	[22]
		Sofosbuvir + daclatasvir for 24 weeks	Yes	[23]

Table 6.1 Hepatitis C virus treatment regimens recommended in treatment-naïve patients with genotypes 1–4, with comparison between EASL and AASLD-IDSA guidelines [5,6,11,14,17–27] (continued overleaf).

Patient group	HCV genotype	EASL guidelines	AASLD-IDSA guidelines	Reference
	4	Sofosbuvir + peg-IFN-α + ribavirin for 12 weeks	Yes, alternative	[19]
		Simeprevir + peg-IFN-α + ribavirin for 12 weeks followed by peg-IFN-α + ribavirin for 12 additional weeks	No	[24]
		Ledipasvir + sofosbuvir + ribavirin for 12 weeks	Yes	[25]
		Paritaprevir/ritonavir/ombitasvir + ribavirin for 24 weeks	Paritaprevir/ ritonavir/ ombitasvir + ribavirin for 12 weeks	[5]
		Simeprevir + sofosbuvir + ribavirin for 12 weeks	No	[14]
		Sofosbuvir + daclatasvir + ribavirin for 12 weeks	No	[20]

Table 6.1 Hepatitis C virus treatment regimens recommended in treatment-naïve patients with genotypes 1–4, with comparison between EASL and AASLD-IDSA guidelines [5,6,11,14,17–27] (continued). 'Yes' denotes that the regimen is recommended, 'Yes, alternative' denotes that it is recommended but as a second-line therapy, 'No' denotes that it is not recommended. Peg-IFN-α, pegylated interferon-alpha.

in patients with HCV genotype 1, these therapies are not endorsed by the AASLD-IDSA guidelines.

A number of IFN-free options are available for patients with chronic HCV genotype 1. The combination of sofosbuvir and ledipasvir in a single tablet formulation administered once daily for 12 weeks is recommended for non-cirrhotic treatment-naïve or treatment-experienced patients, based on SVR rates uniformly above 90% [17,29,30]. In a Phase III, randomized, open-label study by Afdhal et al [30], 440 patients with previous failure to peg-IFN-α-based therapy (including 50–60% previously treated with PI regimens, 45% non-responders, and 20% with cirrhosis) achieved SVR rates of 94% (95% confidence interval [CI] 87–97) after 12 weeks of sofosbuvir and ledipasvir therapy. There was no discontinuation of therapy due to side effects [30]. In patients who received 12 weeks of sofosbuvir, ledipasvir, and ribavirin combination therapy, including patients with cirrhosis, SVR rates were also uniformly high (96% [95% CI 91–99]). EASL guidelines recommend addition of ribavirin to ledipasvir and sofosbuvir in patients with cirrhosis [3] whilst AASLD-IDSA guidelines do not recommend the addition of ribavirin [4]. Importantly, the safety profile of this combination is very favorable, with the most common reported side effects being fatigue, nausea, and headache [30]. Drug interactions are limited to interactions with P-gp inducers, but the combination may be co-administered with all HIV antiretroviral drugs, although, systematic screening should be carried out for potential interactions.

The combination of ombitasvir and paritaprevir boosted with ritonavir and dasabuvir is another IFN-free combination that is effective in patients with HCV genotype 1 infection. Due to differing efficacy in patients with HCV subtype 1a and 1b, it is recommended to treat subtype 1b non-cirrhotic patients for 12 weeks and subtype 1a non-cirrhotic patients for 12 weeks with the addition of ribavirin [3,4,18]. Treatment-experienced non-cirrhotic patients previously treated with peg-IFN-α and ribavirin regimens achieved SVR12 rates of 95–100% [31,32]. Cirrhotic patients with subtype 1b may be treated with this regimen and ribavirin for 12 weeks, but patients with subtype 1a require 24 weeks (SVR12 rates of 99% and 92%, respectively) [3,4,6]. Importantly, in October 2015, the FDA issued a warning regarding the combination of paritaprevir, ritonavir, ombitasvir, and dasabuvir in patients with cirrhosis due to a potential risk of serious liver injury and hepatic decompensation [33]. This recommendation was based on an ongoing adverse events review by the FDA.

Other recommended regimens for patients with genotype 1 include a combination of sofosbuvir and simeprevir for 12 weeks (with the addition of ribavirin in patients with cirrhosis) [14] and sofosbuvir and daclatasvir for 12 weeks (with the addition of ribavirin in patients with cirrhosis). These regimens both demonstrated uniformly high SVR rates in patients with genotype 1:

- Sofosbuvir and simeprevir — patients with METAVIR scores F0–F2 (cohort 1) achieved SVR12 of 92% and patients with METAVIR scores F3–F4 (cohort 2) achieved SVR12 of 94%.
- Daclatasvir and sofosbuvir — patients with subtype 1a achieved SVR12 of 98%, patients with subtype 1b achieved SVR12 of 100%, patients with IL28B CC genotype achieved SVR12 of 93%, and patients with non-CC IL28B genotype achieved SVR12 of 98% [20].

Genotypes 2 and 3

The best option for patients with HCV genotype 2, based on clinical trials, is a combination of sofosbuvir and ribavirin for 12 weeks (or prolonged to 16–20 weeks in patients with cirrhosis). Overall, SVR rates in treatment-naïve non-cirrhotic patients are expected to be greater than 95%, although decline to 88% in treatment-experienced cirrhotic patients treated for only 12 weeks [22]; justifying prolonged therapy in this population [4]. This therapy is generally well tolerated with few side effects. Alternative treatment for patients with cirrhosis and/or treatment-experienced patients infected with HCV genotype 2 includes peg-IFN-α, ribavirin, and sofosbuvir or sofosbuvir and daclatasvir.

Genotype 3 has emerged as one of the difficult-to-treat HCV genotypes in the DAA era [34]. This patient population may be treated with peg-IFN-α, ribavirin, and sofosbuvir for 12 weeks; high SVR rates have been achieved (90–92%), including in treatment-experienced patients and those with cirrhosis, despite a low number of patients being included in studies [21,27]. Alternatively, patients with HCV genotype 3 can be treated with sofosbuvir and daclatasvir for 12 weeks (patients without cirrhosis) or sofosbuvir, daclatasvir, and ribavirin for 24 weeks (patients with cirrhosis) [23].

Genotypes 4, 5, and 6

Genotypes 4, 5, and 6 are less commonly seen, except in certain specific geographic settings (such as the high prevalence of genotype 4 in Egypt). Treatment regimens for genotype 4 are similar to genotype 1, although they generally have been validated in smaller studies [5,14,19,24,25]. For more details please refer to the EASL and AASLD-IDSA guidelines [3,4]. Similarly, genotypes 5 and 6 are less often encountered, at least in Western countries. Recommended regimens include peg-IFN-α, ribavirin, and sofosbuvir for 12 weeks, although the efficacy of this regimen remains unclear in treatment-experienced patients and patients with cirrhosis [19]. Alternatively, the combination of ledipasvir and sofosbuvir for 12 weeks in patients without cirrhosis or ledipasvir, sofosbuvir, and ribavirin for 12 weeks in patients with cirrhosis is recommended; however, data are mostly based on trials in patients with HCV genotype 1 [3,4].

Emerging therapies

A number of newer all-oral, IFN-free regimens may be approved through 2016, some of which are discussed in the following sections.

Velpatasvir and sofosbuvir

The combination of velpatasvir, a second-generation NS5A inhibitor with pan-genotypic activity, and sofosbuvir resulted in high SVR rates of over 90% in patients with genotypes 1, 2, 3, 4, 5, and 6, including patients with previous treatment failure and cirrhosis [35,36]. Even among patients with genotype 3 and cirrhosis who had failed previous therapy, a difficult-to-treat group [31], the SVR rate was 89% compared to 58% in the control sofosbuvir plus ribavirin arm [35]. This combination is also relatively effective in patients with decompensated cirrhosis [37]:

- patients treated with sofosbuvir and velpatasvir for 12 weeks achieved SVR of 83%;
- patients treated with sofosbuvir plus velpatasvir and ribavirin for 12 weeks achieved SVR of 94%; and
- patients treated with sofosbuvir and velpatasvir for 24 weeks achieved SVR 86%.

The side effect profile is also generally favorable with discontinuation rates due to adverse events of less than 1%, [35,36] although, as expected, this rate was slightly higher in patients with decompensated cirrhosis (approximately 3%) [37].

Grazoprevir and elbasvir

A combination of grazoprevir, a second-generation NS3/4A PI, and elbasvir, a NS5A inhibitor, has been found to be promising in difficult-to-treat patients. This combination is a once-daily, single-tablet, IFN-free therapy that has been shown to be highly effective in genotype 1 patients with cirrhosis and previous null responders, with SVR12 rates of greater than 90% [38]. Additionally, the combination of grazoprevir and elbasvir demonstrated an SVR rate of 99% in genotype 1 patients with stage 4–5 chronic kidney disease, a traditionally difficult-to-treat patient population [39].

Management of acute HCV infection

The rate of chronicity after acute HCV infection remains unclear, but is expected to be 50–90% and is higher in asymptomatic patients, males, older patients, and patients with certain genetic polymorphisms, especially near the *interferon-lambda3* gene (*IFNL3*) [40]. Patients with acute HCV infection should be considered for therapy to avoid progression to chronic HCV infection, although, the ideal timeframe for initiation of treatment has not yet been determined. Historically, high SVR rates of greater than 90% were reported with peg-IFN-α monotherapy and EASL guidelines recommend peg-IFN-α monotherapy for 12 weeks (or peg-IFN-α and ribavirin for 24 weeks in patients co-infected with HIV, due to lower SVR rates) [3,41–43]. Despite acknowledging the lack of data, both EASL and AASLD-IDSA also recommend using the relevant DAA-based regimens for chronic HCV infection in patients with acute HCV infection, although further trials are needed to confirm the high SVR rates in this patient population. With the goal to avoid unnecessary treatment in cases of spontaneous HCV viral clearance, the clinician may consider waiting 12–24 weeks after exposure to confirm persistent viral titers before initiating antiviral therapy; however, the level of evidence for this strategy remains low [3,4,41–43]. There is no place for post-exposure prophylaxis with antiviral therapy in the absence of documented HCV transmission, even if the route and time of exposure are known.

Management of HIV/HCV co-infection

The management of patients with HIV/HCV co-infection is similar to that of patients with HCV monoinfection, although, a few specific points must be raised. As discussed, indication for therapy is not dependent on fibrosis stage and all patients should be assessed for therapy with a high priority due to higher rates of disease progression. In addition, numerous complex drug interactions between DAAs and antiretroviral drugs are possible and physicians experienced in the care of both diseases should be consulted before initiation of therapy. In general, drug interactions should be systematically reviewed (for example on www. hep-druginteractions.org) and IFN-free regimens should be favored due to their ease of use and improved tolerability. As of writing, no drug interactions have been reported between sofosbuvir and antiretroviral drugs.

Management of HCV in other patient groups

The treatment of HCV infection in other patient populations, such as patients with severe liver disease, patients awaiting liver transplantation, and patients with HCV recurrence after liver transplantation, remains complex due to potential drug interactions, the lack of data available, and the overall frailty of these patients. In general, these patients should be managed by experienced physicians in centers attached to a liver transplantation unit.

Conclusion

The landscape of antiviral therapy has dramatically evolved over the past years and high SVR rates for most patient groups have been achieved, with reduced side effects. Thus, global eradication of HCV may be achievable within the next few decades; however, this aim may be hampered by the high cost of new drugs that currently limits their use to only those in the highest resource settings. Unfortunately, the high cost of novel therapies will lead to a continued use of suboptimal and more dangerous treatment regimens in developing countries. Therefore, there exists a shift in the field from focusing on medical and technical aspects of HCV eradication to societal and global barriers to eradication, which will be discussed in Chapter 7.

Key points
- All patients with evidence of virological presence of HCV (ie, detectable blood HCV levels) should be assessed for possible antiviral therapy.
- The highest priority for therapy is assigned to patients with HCV at highest risk of developing complications, including patients with METAVIR stage F3 fibrosis or cirrhosis, liver transplant recipients, and patients with severe extrahepatic manifestations.

- Guidelines for HCV antiviral therapy are rapidly evolving and the clinician must review the most updated guidelines prior to introducing antiviral therapy.
- Most patients will be candidates for IFN-free DAA-based therapy.

References

1   Girardin F, Goossens N, Vernaz N, Negro F. [Rethinking the reimbursement policy of direct acting antivirals against chronic hepatitis C]. *Rev Med Suisse*. 2015;11:1610–1612, 1614–1616.

2   van der Meer AJ, Veldt BJ, Feld JJ, et al. Association between sustained virological response and all-cause mortality among patients with chronic hepatitis C and advanced hepatic fibrosis. *JAMA*. 2012;308:2584–2593.

3   European Association for Study of Liver. EASL Recommendations on Treatment of Hepatitis C 2015. *J Hepatol*. 2015;63:199–236.

4   AASLD/IDSA HCV Guidance Panel. Hepatitis C guidance: AASLD-IDSA recommendations for testing, managing, and treating adults infected with hepatitis C virus. *Hepatology*. 2015;62:932–954.

5   Hézode C, Asselah T, Reddy KR, et al. Ombitasvir plus paritaprevir plus ritonavir with or without ribavirin in treatment-naive and treatment-experienced patients with genotype 4 chronic hepatitis C virus infection (PEARL-I): a randomised, open-label trial. *Lancet*. 2015;385:2502–2509.

6   Poordad F, Hezode C, Trinh R, et al, ABT-450/r-ombitasvir and dasabuvir with ribavirin for hepatitis C with cirrhosis. *N Eng J Med*. 2014;370:1973–1982.

7   European Association for Study of Liver. EASL Clinical Practice Guidelines: management of hepatitis C virus infection. *J Hepatol*. 2011;55:245–264.

8   Manns MP, Wedemeyer H, CornbergM. Treating viral hepatitis C: efficacy, side effects, and complications. *Gut*. 2006;55:1350–1359.

9   Jacobson IM, McHutchison JG, Dusheiko G, et al. Telaprevir for previously untreated chronic hepatitis C virus infection. *N Eng J Med*. 2011;364:2405–2416.

10   Poordad F, McCone J Jr, Bacon BR, et al. Boceprevir for untreated chronic HCV genotype 1 infection. *N Eng J Med*. 2011;364:1195–1206.

11   Jacobson IM, Dore GJ, Foster GR, et al. Simeprevir with pegylated interferon alfa 2a plus ribavirin in treatment-naive patients with chronic hepatitis C virus genotype 1 infection (QUEST-1): a phase 3, randomised, double-blind, placebo-controlled trial. *Lancet*. 2014;384:403–413.

12   Manns M, Marcellin P, Poordad F, et al. Simeprevir with pegylated interferon alfa 2a or 2b plus ribavirin in treatment-naive patients with chronic hepatitis C virus genotype 1 infection (QUEST-2): a randomised, double-blind, placebo-controlled phase 3 trial. *Lancet*. 2014;384:414–426.

13   Zeuzem S, Berg T, Gane E, et al. Simeprevir increases rate of sustained virologic response among treatment-experienced patients with HCV genotype-1 infection: a phase IIb trial. *Gastroenterology*. 2013;146:430–441.

14   Lawitz E, Sulkowski MS, Ghalib R, et al. Simeprevir plus sofosbuvir, with or without ribavirin, to treat chronic infection with hepatitis C virus genotype 1 in non-responders to pegylated interferon and ribavirin and treatment-naive patients: the COSMOS randomised study. *Lancet*. 2014;384:1756–1765.

15   Kwo P, Gitlin N, Nahass R, et al. LP14: A Phase 3, randomised, open-label study to evaluate the efficacy and safety of 8 and 12 weeks of simeprevir (SMV) plus sofosbuvir (SOF) in treatment-naïve and -experienced patients with chronic HCV genotype 1 infection without cirrhosis: Optimist-1. *J Hepatol*. 2015;62 (Suppl 2):S270.

16 Fontaine H, Lazarus A, Pol S, et al. Bradyarrhythmias associated with sofosbuvir treatment. *N Eng J Med*. 2015;373:1886–1888.

17 Kowdley KV, Gordon SC, Reddy KR, et al. Ledipasvir and sofosbuvir for 8 or 12 weeks for chronic HCV without cirrhosis. *N Eng J Med*. 2014;370:1879–1888.

18 Feld JJ, Kowdley KV, Coakley E, et al. Treatment of HCV with ABT-450/r-ombitasvir and dasabuvir with ribavirin. *N Eng J Med*. 2014;370:1594–1603.

19 Lawitz E, Mangia A, Wyles D, et al. Sofosbuvir for previously untreated chronic hepatitis C infection. *N Engl J Med*. 2013;368:1878–1887.

20 Sulkowski MS, Gardiner DF, Rodriguez-Torres M, et al. Daclatasvir plus sofosbuvir for previously treated or untreated chronic HCV infection. *N Eng J Med*. 2014;370:211–221.

21 Lawitz E, Lalezari JP, Hassanein T, et al. Sofosbuvir in combination with peginterferon alfa-2a and ribavirin for non-cirrhotic, treatment-naive patients with genotypes 1, 2, and 3 hepatitis C infection: a randomised, double-blind, phase 2 trial. *Lancet Infect Dis*. 2013;13:401–408.

22 Zeuzem S, Dusheiko GM, Salupere, et al. Sofosbuvir and ribavirin in HCV genotypes 2 and 3. *N Eng J Med*. 2014;370:1993–2001.

23 Nelson DR, Cooper JN, Lalezari JP, et al. All-oral 12-week treatment with daclatasvir plus sofosbuvir in patients with hepatitis C virus genotype 3 infection: ALLY-3 phase III study. *Hepatology*. 2015;61:1127–1135.

24 Moreno C, Hezode C, Marcellin P, et al. Efficacy and safety of simeprevir with PegIFN/ribavirin in naïve or experienced patients infected with chronic HCV genotype 4. *J Hepatol*. 2015;62:1047–1055.

25 Kohli A, Kapoor R, Sims Z, et al. Ledipasvir and sofosbuvir for hepatitis C genotype 4: a proof-of-concept, single-centre, open-label phase 2a cohort study. *Lancet Infect Dis*. 2015;15:1049–1054.

26 Jacobson IM, Gordon SC, Kowdley KV, et al. Sofosbuvir for hepatitis C genotype 2 or 3 in patients without treatment options. *N Engl J Med*. 2013;368:1867–1877.

27 Lawitz E, Poordad F, Brainard DM, et al. Sofosbuvir with peginterferon-ribavirin for 12 weeks in previously treated patients with hepatitis C genotype 2 or 3 and cirrhosis. *Hepatology*. 2015;61:769–775.

28 Jensen DM, O'Leary J, Pockros P, et al. Safety and efficacy of sofosbuvir-containing regimens for hepatitis C: real-world experience in a diverse, longitudinal observational cohort. Abstract presented at: 65th Annual Meeting of the American Association for the Study of Liver Diseases; November 7–11, 2014; Boston, US.

29 Afdhal N, Zeuzem S, Kwo P, et al. Ledipasvir and sofosbuvir for untreated HCV genotype 1 infection. *N Eng J Med*. 2014;370:1889–1898.

30 Afdhal N, Reddy KR, Nelson DR, et al. Ledipasvir and sofosbuvir for previously treated HCV genotype 1 infection. *N Eng J Med*. 2014;370:1483–1493.

31 Andreone P, Colombo MG, Enejosa JV, et al. ABT-450, ritonavir, ombitasvir, and dasabuvir achieves 97% and 100% sustained virologic response with or without ribavirin in treatment-experienced patients with HCV genotype 1b infection. *Gastroenterology*. 2014;147:359–365.

32 Zeuzem S, Jacobson IM, Baykal T, et al. Retreatment of HCV with ABT-450/r-ombitasvir and dasabuvir with ribavirin. *N Engl J Med*. 2014;370:1604–1614.

33 US Food and Drug Administration website. FDA Drug Safety Communication: FDA warns of serious liver injury risk with hepatitis C treatments Viekira Pak and Technivie. www.fda.gov/Drugs/DrugSafety/ucm468634.htm. Updated Oct 22, 2015. Accessed Feb 11, 2015.

34 Goossens N, Negro F. Is genotype 3 of the hepatitis C virus the new villain? *Hepatology*. 2014;59:2403–2412.

35 Foster GR, Afdhal N, Roberts SK, et al. Sofosbuvir and Velpatasvir for HCV Genotype 2 and 3 Infection. *N Engl J Med*. 2015;373:2608–2617

36 Feld JJ, Jacobson IM, Hézode C, et al. Sofosbuvir and Velpatasvir for HCV Genotype 1, 2, 4, 5, and 6 Infection. *N Engl J Med*. 2015;373:2599–2607.

37   Curry MP, O'Leary JG, Bzowej N, et al. Sofosbuvir and velpatasvir for HCV in patients with decompensated cirrhosis. *N Engl J Med*. 2015;373:2618–2628.

38   Lawitz E, Gane E, Pearlman B, et al. Efficacy and safety of 12 weeks versus 18 weeks of treatment with grazoprevir (MK-5172) and elbasvir (MK-8742) with or without ribavirin for hepatitis C virus genotype 1 infection in previously untreated patients with cirrhosis and patients with previous null response with or without cirrhosis (C-WORTHY): a randomised, open-label phase 2 trial. *Lancet*. 2015;385:1075–1086.

39   Roth D, Nelson DR, Bruchfeld A, et al. Grazoprevir plus elbasvir in treatment-naive and treatment-experienced patients with hepatitis C virus genotype 1 infection and stage 4-5 chronic kidney disease (the C-SURFER study): a combination phase 3 study. *Lancet*. 2015;386:1537–1545.

40   Negro F. Hepatitis C virus epidemiology, pathogenesis, diagnosis, and natural history. In: Zeuzem S, Afdhal NH, ed. *inPractice Hepatology*. 2015. www.inpractice.com/Textbooks/Hepatology.aspx. Updated July 24, 2015. Accessed Feb 11, 2016.

41   Gerlach JT, Diepolder HM, Zachoval R, et al. Acute hepatitis C: high rate of both spontaneous and treatment-induced viral clearance. *Gastroenterology*. 2003;125:80–88.

42   Santantonio T, Wiegand J, Gerlach JT. Acute hepatitis C: current status and remaining challenges. *J Hepatol*. 2008;49:625–633.

43   Corey KE, Mendez-Navarro J, Gorospe EC, Zheng H, Chung RT. Early treatment improves outcomes in acute hepatitis C virus infection: a meta-analysis. *J Viral Hepat*. 2010;17:201–207.

Chapter 7

Future challenges

The recent development of very efficient antiviral drugs (Chapter 6) that can potentially cure virtually all treated patients, without clinically significant side effects, has opened new perspectives for the global management of hepatitis C. The eradication of hepatitis C virus (HCV) infection from entire swathes of land, if not worldwide, has been evocated, and the ongoing national treatment program put in place in Georgia — if proven successful — may provide the proof of concept regarding the feasibility of this strategy [1]. However, if many barriers to universal treatment access have disappeared (eg, treatment-emerging adverse events and the fear of them that prevented many patients and care providers from administering IFN-α-containing regimens until recently) new compelling challenges have emerged that will be briefly discussed in this conclusive chapter.

The first concept that has been emphasized in recent modelizations is the fact that the current treatment uptake is, in most countries, insufficient to significantly impact future morbidity and mortality related to HCV, even after factoring in the higher efficacy of direct acting antiviral (DAA)-based regimens [2]. Thus, in order to reduce the mortality by 90% by 2030, ie, when the peak of the HCV-related health burden is expected to be reached in most developed countries [3], the treatment uptake should be multiplied by a factor of ~4 in many countries. This issue alone poses two problems:

1. setting up and following antiviral treatment in so many patients would require the participation of general practitioners to national

© Springer International Publishing Switzerland 2016   79
N. Goossens et al. (eds.), *Handbook of Hepatitis C*,
DOI 10.1007/978-3-319-28053-0_7

campaigns, and even though current treatments are simpler educational programs would be crucial; and

2. more importantly, treating more patients depends on increased diagnosis rates.

Historically, risk-based screening strategies have proven unsuccessful [4], and in most countries the proportion of undiagnosed, infected persons remains high (on average ~50%). For this reason, alternative approaches have been proposed in recent years, such as the birth cohort screening strategy. In the US, persons born between 1945 and 1964 (the so-called 'baby boomers') account for 27% of the general population but as many as 76.5% of all HCV infected persons [5]. Thus, it has been estimated that testing (and successfully treating) all infected 'baby boomers' for HCV, irrespective of risk factors would avoid 47,189 more cases of hepatocellular carcinoma (HCC), 15,484 more liver transplants, and 120,879 deaths than a conventional risk-based screening strategy [5]. Whether this strategy will be successful remains to be proven, but it is clear that unless more patients are identified who can be treated, the benefit of a widespread implementation of DAA-based therapy will be lower than expected.

Treating more patients will involve serious logistic issues, but the most important challenge posed by new DAAs is the market price. When sofosbuvir was first licensed in the US, a full 12-week course cost in excess of 80,000 USD, and more recent antivirals are just as expensive. Universal treatment with DAA would involve prohibitive costs even for resource-rich countries, and new pricing models that reconcile fair and equitable access to effective drugs, with profitability for the drug makers, are urgently needed. Regulatory authorities have reacted to high prices with severe restrictions on drug use, eg, by limiting the access of DAAs to patients with advanced fibrosis, clinically significant extrahepatic manifestations, or in the setting of liver transplantation. These limitations are difficult to accept from the ethical standpoint. Treatment may reasonably be indicated also in situations other than those characterized by a severe liver disease, including patients at high risk of transmission (eg, intravenous drug users or HIV-infected men who have sex with men), fertile women planning a pregnancy, or patients with invalidating fatigue (that severely affects daily life and/or social interactions).

The advent of shorter duration regimens may also help in this respect, especially for patients with mild disease [6].

Additional issues that require further research concern the management of resistance-associated variants (RAVs), especially those affording resistance to NS5A inhibitors (eg, Q30R and Y93H), and the need for a vaccine. Eradication via universal immunization would theoretically be possible, given the fact that there are no animal reservoirs of HCV. However, developing a cross-reactive immunity to HCV has proven an enormous challenge. Recent approaches based on T cell immunity targeting conserved viral epitopes seem promising and may circumvent the technical shortcomings encountered until now [7,8].

Finally, what can still be expected from translational research in the field of HCV pathobiology? The study of the HCV–host interactions has provided a wealth of information that may be useful to improve not only our knowledge of liver cell biology, but also of the mechanisms of diseases other than hepatitis C. To give a simple example, the recent findings that HCV causes insulin resistance via endocrine mechanisms, ie, based on a hitherto unsuspected liver-muscle crosstalk [9,10], has provided a stimulating model that may help with understanding the pathogenesis of type 2 diabetes. Unravelling other mechanisms of disease, such as liver fibrogenesis and oncogenesis, may still depend on experimental models exploiting HCV. For this reason, it is important that HCV research remains alive, even at a time when we may see the end of the global pandemic of hepatitis C.

Key points
- Many of the traditional barriers to treatment have disappeared (eg, adverse side effects to antiviral drugs), but new barriers have emerged.
- The advent of highly efficacious DAAs has revolutionized treatment (allowing shorter regimens and significantly reducing the burden of adverse events); however, uptake of treatment is still insufficient to impact on the morbidity and mortality of hepatitis C virus.

- Economic and societal issues are being faced due to the high market prices of new therapies, leaving even resource-rich countries unable to provide treatment for every person with hepatitis C infection.
- To support increased uptake of treatment, national campaigns must be enforced and diagnosis rates must increase.
- The emergence of resistance must be managed, which is a particular problem with NS5A inhibitors.
- Development of vaccines could potentially lead to eradication of disease, but development of cross-reactive immunity is an enormous challenge.

References

Printed in the United States
By Bookmasters